W9-ACF-230

Successful Administration of Senior Housing

To my children, Kate, Liz, and Sarah,
whose love makes our house a home

Successful Administration of Senior Housing
Working with Elderly Residents

Nancy W. Sheehan

SAGE Publications
International Educational and Professional Publisher
Newbury Park   London   New Delhi

For information address:

SAGE Publications, Inc.
2455 Teller Road
Newbury Park, California 91320

SAGE Publications Ltd.
6 Bonhill Street
London EC2A 4PU
United Kingdom

SAGE Publications India Pvt. Ltd.
M-32 Market
Greater Kailash I
New Delhi 110 048 India

Printed in the United States of America

Library of Congress Cataloging-in-Publication Data

Sheehan, Nancy W.
    Successful administration of senior housing: working with elderly residents / Nancy W. Sheehan.
        p. cm.
    Includes bibliographical references (p.   ) and index.
    ISBN 0-8039-4524-8. — ISBN 0-8039-4525-6 (pbk.)
    1. Old age homes—United States—Management. 2. Aged—Housing—United States—Management. 3. Social work with the aged.—United States. 4. Aged—Home care—United States—Management. I. Title.
HV1454.2.U6S54   1992
363.5 '946'068—dc20   92-18609

92 93 94 95 10 9 8 7 6 5 4 3 2 1

Sage Production Editor: Diane S. Foster

Contents

Foreword

CONSIDERING that at least 2.5 million Americans live in housing explicitly planned for and occupied by people over age 60 or so, it is astonishing that this century of population aging has had to wait 92 years for the appearance of Dr. Sheehan's book. A less hyperbolic statement would date the high perceived salience of housing for older people from about 1959, but the years since that time have seen extraordinary concern for many facets of planned housing. National, state, and local levels, the governmental, non-profit, and for-profit sectors, policy specialists, planners, designers, and researchers are some of the interest groups that have given major attention to this form of service for the elderly population. Service planners and deliverers have also recognized housing as an essential component of the total community service system.

For some reason, however, housing as real estate (number of units), housing as a physical entity (designing for human needs), housing as a haven (physical security), and other images have dominated our concerns. Relatively absent has been the concept of housing as "care management," a term used by James Sykes and elaborated as the overriding topic of Dr. Sheehan's book. Although many of us who have been active in supporting the growth of quality housing programs have bemoaned the neglect of housing administration as a developing profession, few attempts to fill the gap have appeared. One must, of course, acknowledge some concrete efforts that have been made to upgrade the quality of housing management through training programs. The American Association of Homes for the Aged has led the way for many years in providing seminars, instructional material, and certification guidelines for nonprofit management. The Real Estate Institute has shown some similar interest, and the National Center for Housing Management has valiantly attempted to provide training for people already engaged in management, but less rich in the care aspects of management.

The absence of a source such as the present book may well have been a major factor in limiting the development of care management to a level equal to that of fiscal and administrative management. Very literally this is the first book ever written that attempts to apply the large body of knowledge in gerontology to the task of person-oriented housing administration. Compare this lack to the long list of books on housing policy and housing planning or design that has appeared over the past few decades. One of the problems is the contrast between the glitter of the physical housing and the intangibility of management. Few housing administrators have become heroes. It seems very likely, however, that Dr. Sheehan's book will have a hand in creating some such heroes.

The reader will find the book informed by the last word in gerontological theory and research, integrated so successfully that one is aware primarily of the good sense displayed in the discussion of each of her topics. A real strength is her willingness to acknowledge the complexity of the issues she discusses. No person will experience a sense of unreality as he or she compares real management issues with the thoughtful suggestions advanced here. Effective administrative skills will become enhanced through the feelings of confidence engendered by Dr. Sheehan's acknowledgment of common problems and by the concrete suggestions offered for handling them.

In particular, there are many areas in which positive control may be exercised by the administrator. Decisions regarding occupancy, orienting new tenants, monitoring the match between tenant need and what the housing can provide, fostering positive social attitudes and behaviors, enriching on-site housing programs, adapting the physical environment to individual needs, and relating the housing context to the external community of neighbors, family, and formal services are only a few of the topics discussed. Despite the clear suggestions made for applying knowledge to such problems, the overall philosophy of respect for tenant autonomy comes through at every step. The housing manager is ideally an effective partner of the tenant, not the expert who always knows best.

Although many of these topics have been discussed in scattered literature, one section of her book provides material that is brand new and timely. As an expert in mental health and developmental disability, Dr. Sheehan has something new to say about dealing with the mental health of older tenants. Alcohol abuse, mental illness, mental retardation, and physical handicap, as well as possible age integration, are realities of the present-day housing scene. The Section 504 legislation of access and other more recent regulations specify the right of people with all types of disability to be accommodated in publicly assisted housing. The suggestion as to how management can deal with these admittedly difficult problems are fortified by first-hand knowledge of local programs that have successfully coped with integration of disabled and "mainstream" elders.

A last thought is the hope that enhanced management expertise can help us survive what are surely the darkest days yet seen in the history of housing for the elders. The United States has endured a full decade of famine in planned housing for any but the most economically privileged elders. Every program except the Section 202 program has either stopped completely (e.g., new public housing construction) or has been pure political tokenism (e.g., the Congregate Housing Services Program or the Congregate Voucher Program). Existing housing is being starved in maintenance, rehabilitation, and service-support funding, despite the clear evidence that the aging-in-place population is straining the limits of such environments to meet its needs. A crisis of need and demand is certain to come in the last decade of the twentieth century.

The lack of national economic resources is the obvious excuse given for such neglect. It will probably be several more years before the crisis deepens enough and political ideology moves enough to enable the nation to accept a realistic level of taxation and public-private partnership to reverse the neglect. In the meantime, creative, effective housing management may be our only hope. The silver lining of the housing neglect of the 1980s may be that there will finally be motivation to utilize management resources to their fullest potential. Creating good management out of hunger is a bad rationale for it, but if creative management achieves its momentum during a period of starvation, it should flourish extraordinarily well when housing resources in general improve.

M. POWELL LAWTON, PH.D.
Philadelphia Geriatric Center

Acknowledgments

I am indebted to so many people who provided inspiration, help, and encouragement as I have pursued my interest in senior housing. The Applied Fellowship Program of the Gerontological Society of America and the Connecticut Department on Aging provided funding for my initial experience doing research in senior housing. From this early experience, I am particularly indebted to Kevin Mahoney, Ph.D., for his guidance and support in helping me learn about applied research. I am also indebted to the many elderly tenants in public senior housing who openly shared their experiences concerning living in senior housing.

Other research endeavors examining facets of planned housing environments have been made possible with the support and cooperation of housing agencies throughout the state. The Connecticut Department of Housing, Connecticut Housing Finance Agency, and local housing authorities have provided consistent support and encouragement in facilitating research examining senior housing. Among the individuals who have made these partnerships possible are Michael Duffy and Richard LoPresti, Connecticut Department of Housing, Ralph Cheyney and Bette Meyerson, Connecticut Housing Finance Agency, and Horace McCaulley, Connecticut Department on Aging.

In addition, the Administration on Aging, U.S. Department of Health and Human Services, has provided funding to carry out several model projects addressing the needs of older persons in senior housing. Both the Elderly Renters Project (90AT042501) and the Elderly Supportive Services Program (90AM043901) have provided the opportunity to work with many dedicated people working the fields of both aging and elderly housing. I am deeply indebted to the many people who have shared their knowledge, expertise, and skills in working with tenants in senior housing. The idea for this book grew out of the experiences of the Elderly Renters Project designed to train housing managers and social services providers to work with elderly tenants. This book is an attempt to address the complex issues that housing managers and social service providers identified growing out of their work with elderly tenants.

Finally, without the help and technical assistance of my husband, Alfred Tufano, I would never have been able to complete this project. His tireless help in editing versions of the manuscript has provided the essential support and encouragement that I needed.

1

Introduction

Ironically, they wouldn't cause so many problems if we didn't care. If we were just a landlord or just interested in collecting their money, it would really be no problem. But, there is that commitment and that's where you become involved with the residents. . . . You get to like George. He's 91 years old and you can see his health is failing. You like the guy. You know he doesn't want to leave. How do you tell him he has to go? You can't. You try and work it so that he can stay here as long as possible.

Apartment Manager of Elderly Housing
(Wolfsen, Barker, & Mitteness, 1990, pp. 109-110)

THIS book is written for housing managers, social service providers, health care professionals, and gerontologists who work with frail elderly tenants in senior housing. The term "senior housing" includes any type of planned housing intended to serve independent older persons. Using this definition, the book is written for professionals working with elderly tenants who reside in a variety of age-segregated independent housing settings. These include federal public senior housing, federally assisted housing, retirement

1

communities, and state-subsidized elderly housing (U.S. Senate Special Committee on Aging, 1990). The book addresses one of the major problems involved in senior housing—how to meet the increased support needs of elderly tenants in housing environments that lack adequate supportive services.

PURPOSE OF THIS BOOK

This book provides information and concrete strategies that may prove helpful in responding to the needs of elderly tenants with disabilities. The information presented throughout this book is drawn from a variety of different sources. Some chapters draw heavily from information derived from the fields of gerontology, housing management, public policy, and demography, which directly relate to elderly housing. Other chapters are based upon the knowledge and expertise of housing managers and other professionals who have developed successful strategies and tools for working with elderly tenants.

The purpose of the book is to give a better understanding of the problems that older persons experience in senior housing, an increased awareness of management strategies and tools to respond to frailty among elderly tenants, and a better understanding of the linkage between the housing management role and ways of serving elderly tenants. In addition it will give professionals an increased awareness of the importance of collaboration among housing managers, social service providers, and health care professionals to more effectively and humanely serve the needs of vulnerable elderly renters with disabilities.

Senior Housing: More Than Shelter

Since the late 1960s there have been growing efforts to define senior housing as more than shelter alone. These efforts have focused on expanding the view of senior housing beyond the earlier "bricks and mortar" approach to include recognition of the support needs of elderly tenants. The rationale for this expanded view was based upon the assumption that elderly tenants represent a vulnerable or "at risk" group due to the normal dependencies of aging (Benedict, 1977; Thompson, 1982).

Much less attention, however, has focused on the mechanisms for providing services in senior housing and the role of housing managers within this expanded view. To date, housing managers have received little concrete help or assistance from housing experts, public policymakers, or gerontologists concerning how to address the support needs of elderly tenants or how to manage the complex problems and issues that emerge as elderly tenants experience increased needs for supportive services. As traditional senior housing accommodates more and more dependent elderly tenants, the interest in independent housing as more than just a place to live will dramatically increase.

Aging in Place in Senior Housing

Aging in place in senior housing refers to the phenomenon that growing numbers of elderly tenants have resided in their age-segregated independent apartment units for 10 to 15 years or more. These tenants, who moved into independent senior housing when they were in their 60s and 70s, are now well into their 80s, 90s, and beyond. One of the major consequences of aging in place is the increased risk of functional impairment associated with advancing age.

Many of the longest-living tenants in senior housing experience multiple physical, social, and psychological aging-related changes that result in moderate to severe impairments, limiting their ability to live independently in the community. As a result, many tenants who have aged in place require help or assistance in carrying out the necessary activities of daily living. In response, housing professionals and social service providers increasingly are called upon to meet the support needs of growing numbers of elderly tenants.

Evidence of the aging in place phenomenon is demonstrated in the changing age profile of senior housing tenants. Both the numbers and percentages of tenants in senior housing who are now in their 80s and 90s have dramatically increased. It is common for many senior housing complexes to house large numbers of tenants in their 80s. While estimates vary, as a rule between one quarter to one third of the tenants in senior housing are 80 years of age and older (Sheehan & Mahoney, 1984; U.S. House of Representatives Select Committee on Aging, 1989). The shift in the age profile of senior housing complexes is most apparent in older federally assisted housing complexes that have been in operation 15 or 20 years (U.S. House of Representatives Select Committee on Aging, 1989).

In addition to aging in place, a second, much less frequently considered factor has contributed to the "aging" of senior housing complexes—the ages of tenants entering the complex (Lawton, Greenbaum, & Liebowitz, 1980). New tenants entering senior housing are moving in at significantly older ages. Consequently, as a result of both aging in place and the ages of "new" residents, the tenant population in senior housing is dramatically "aging."

Because the likelihood of functional impairment increases with age, particularly after age 75, the "aging" of senior housing complexes has brought about significant changes in the numbers of elderly tenants who are no longer self-sufficient in their ability to carry out the necessary tasks of daily living. Estimates indicate that among persons 85 years of age and older between one third and one half need support from others to carry out either basic activities of daily living (bathing, grooming, dressing, etc.) or instrumental activities of daily living (transportation, shopping, housekeeping, etc.) (National Center for Health Statistics, 1986; U.S. Department of Health and Human Services, 1987). As the prevalence of functional impairment increases, senior housing managers and social service professionals struggle to find innovative ways to respond to both the support needs of individual elderly tenants and the increased support needs of "aging" senior housing populations as a whole.

Meeting the Needs of Elderly Tenants in Senior Housing

The challenges of working with elderly senior housing tenants whose ability to care for themselves is impaired are in many ways similar to those involved in working with any community-living older person with disabilities. There are important differences, however, that social service and health care professionals need to consider in developing care plans. Senior housing tenants, as a group, evidence more risk factors that threaten their continued ability to live independently than do other groups of community-living elderly. More specifically, senior housing tenants are poorer, more likely to be single, more likely to live alone, suffer more limitations in their functional ability, have more limited informal support networks, and experience a greater risk of nursing home placement than other groups of elderly (Morris, Gutkin, Ruchlin, & Sherwood, 1990; Schlesinger & Morris, 1982). The greater vulnerability of senior housing tenants is frequently overlooked by social service and health care professionals. In fact many social service providers and health care professionals assume that the tenants in senior housing are "better off" than other groups of community-living elderly (Sheehan, 1986b). As a result, in communities where the availability of formal support services is limited, services are not targeted to senior housing tenants.

Numerous factors, however, create obstacles in meeting the needs of "aging" senior housing tenants. First, since senior housing complexes were built for independent elderly, there are no established mechanisms or procedures for providing support services to assist elderly tenants. In fact, senior housing complexes that provide supportive services to elderly tenants do so by piecing together whatever services are available in the local community. This method of service delivery has recently been described as the CACC ("Catch as Catch Can") approach. Second, when most senior housing complexes were initially constructed, cost factors and related design decisions limited the available space to be used for adding on-site support services as the functional capacity of tenants decreased. As a result, few senior housing complexes have adequate space to house social service or health professionals to respond to the emerging needs of elderly tenants. Third, community-based residential alternatives to senior housing that provide more supportive services are generally not available. As tenants experience increased frailty, their sole residential option is often a nursing home. For most impaired elderly tenants, fear of nursing home placement makes this an unacceptable alternative. Pressures build on housing managers to maintain the most frail tenants to avoid nursing home placement. Finally, the attitudes of professionals who view senior housing tenants as "better off" limit efforts to target services to elderly senior housing tenants.

**Senior Housing Managers and Social
Service Professionals as Pioneers**

Housing managers and social service providers confronting the problems of frailty and dependence among senior housing tenants are pioneers in responding to the challenge of aging in place in senior housing. With little help or direction from public policy-makers or housing experts, they are charting new directions for senior housing in response to the "aging" of tenants. Among the challenges that they confront are:

1. What is the appropriate response to increasing frailty among elderly senior housing tenants?
2. How can the complex problems of vulnerable or at risk elderly tenants be effectively evaluated and assessed to determine when the independent housing environment is no longer appropriate for an impaired tenant?
3. What specific guidelines are available to help define the new role of housing manager with the expanded view of senior housing?
4. What support is available to protect the quality of life for all elderly tenants?
5. What community-based services are available to assist vulnerable tenants in living "independently" in the community?

Throughout the chapters of this book these and other issues confronting housing managers, social service providers, and health care professionals will be addressed.

OVERVIEW

Each of the chapters in this book presents critical issues that influence the quality of life of elderly senior housing tenants and suggested strategies for working with elderly tenants. Information is derived from research, practice models, and case studies that increase our understanding of the complex dynamic interactions that occur in senior housing. The material that will follow discusses sociocultural, theoretical, and applied perspectives that affect efforts to meet the needs of elderly tenants.

The remainder of this introductory chapter describes a person-environment transactional model to help organize the information presented in the book. The model provides insight into the multiple influences operating in senior housing and how these factors interact to affect the changes that occur. The transactional model helps to integrate diverse information about health, functional impairment, mobility, management style and skills, sociohistorical trends, physical design, and social influences to understand both stability and change in senior housing. Among the critical factors discussed are tenant characteristics, social support systems, residential policies and programs, physical setting, staff attitudes, and social climate.

Chapter 2, "Significant Trends Affecting Senior Housing," highlights the most significant factors that have altered our thinking about senior housing. From the perspective of practitioners, this information gives the context in which the more practical suggestions and strategies emerge. The background material is intended not only to help the reader understand earlier influences that have shaped thinking about senior housing, but also to anticipate some of the changes that will occur over the next 20 years.

Chapters 3 through 11 provide both theoretical and practical information concerning what professionals should know for successful work with elderly tenants. The failure of housing experts and gerontologists to address systematically the complex issues involved in managing elderly housing is indicated in only a "patchwork" of information that is available. These chapters attempt to synthesize available information that affects work with elderly tenants.

Chapter 3, "The Changing Role of Housing Manager: Redefining the Role and Responsibilities of Housing Managers," examines who the managers of elderly housing are, how managing senior housing is different from managing other types of housing, efforts to define the changing role and responsibilities of housing managers in response to the "aging" of senior housing tenants, the concept of housing manager as "care manager," and how conceptions of autonomy impact on interactions with elderly tenants.

Chapter 4, "Management Practices and Policies and Aging in Place," discusses how policies and procedures in senior housing contribute to successful management and impact on the quality of life of older tenants. Particular attention is focused on the importance of screening, admission, and relocation policies for managing senior housing. The remainder of the chapter examines the importance of assessment in working with vulnerable elderly tenants. A number of assessment tools and strategies for evaluating elderly tenants are discussed.

Chapter 5, "Physical Design and Quality of Life in Senior Housing," examines how aspects of the physical environment influence elderly tenants' ability to live independently in housing that maximizes social and functional competencies. Suggestions for modifying physical and design characteristics to enhance tenant competence are discussed.

Chapter 6, "Building a Positive Social Environment in Senior Housing," discusses the dimensions of the social environment in senior housing, strategies for empowering elderly tenants and fostering a positive social climate, and the influence of residential factors (policies, planned services, and tenant and staff characteristics) on the social environment. Specific attention focuses on the relationship between loneliness and social activity and the importance of planned social activities for achieving social goals and improving the quality of life among elderly residents.

Chapter 7, "Social Support in the Lives of Elderly Tenants," takes a closer look at the importance of social support in the lives of elderly tenants and the consequences of positive and negative social support and interaction for elderly tenants' well-being. Ways for working with family members, tenants, and quasi-formal support systems to enhance informal support are discussed.

Chapter 8, "Formal Services in Senior Housing," examines the role of formal services in providing needed assistance to elderly tenants. Particular attention is focused on targeting services to at risk elderly tenants, networking, and innovative service delivery programs developed in senior housing.

Chapter 9, "Special Mental Health Issues in Senior Housing," highlights other challenging issues in senior housing, including alcoholism and alcohol abuse among elderly residents, cognitive impairment, and depression. Strategies for identifying the nature of problems are discussed.

Chapter 10, "Working With Special Populations in Senior Housing," explores the integration of persons with developmental disabilities and chronic mental impairment into senior housing. Specific attention focuses on the implications of Fair Housing legislation for housing managers and their management of senior housing, stereotypes, and prejudices directed against persons with disabilities, and strategies for working with special populations.

The final chapter, "Housing Managers, Social Service Providers, and Health Care Professionals Working Together," describes the need for housing professionals, social services providers, and health care professionals to work together to address the complex problems of elderly tenants. Recognizing the areas of potential conflict that divide housing, social service and health care professionals, this chapter attempts to develop an empathetic understanding of the respective roles of professionals involved with elderly tenants and strategies for overcoming barriers that prevent cooperation. As we look to senior housing in the year 2000 and beyond, the need for these partnerships will increase. The implications of future demographic changes for meeting the needs of senior housing tenants are discussed.

FRAMEWORK: PERSON-ENVIRONMENT TRANSACTIONS

Because the phenomenon of aging in place reflects *both* changes in resident competence and changes in the environment, those working with elderly residents should understand how the person and the environment are interdependent. To underscore the importance of the complex changes that occur in elderly housing, the overall framework for the book draws upon a transactional model of person-environment interaction. Unlike other environmental models in which the environment and the person exist as separate entities, the transactional model assumes that the environment and the person are interdependent. Neither the environment nor the person exists as a separate entity, rather, each element derives its meaning from the other. Thus, according to Moore (1986), "person and environment are defined in the context of each other and in the context of the events that bind the two together in space and time" (p. 2). Efforts to understand a particular phenomenon or behavior cannot treat the person or the environment in isolation, rather, the person must be defined in relation to the environment in which he or she exists. Several concrete examples help to illustrate how the person and environment are mutually defined. Using the concept of competence, an individual's competence cannot be defined without reference to a particular environment. A highly competent American who is able to effectively communicate all of his or her needs becomes impaired when traveling to a foreign country where he or she does not speak the native tongue and no one speaks English. Similarly, an astronaut who is capable of complete independent functioning when on earth experiences functional limitations when operating in space (Faletti, 1984). In another instance, an elderly tenant's ability to function independently is partly defined by the individual's familiarity with the environment. Familiarity with a particular environment enhances the individual's competence by increasing the amount of control that he or she can achieve (Lawton, 1985). Each example underscores the basic assumption that the person and environment are interdependent and rely on each other for meaning.

According to the transactional model, change (i.e., in functional level, decreased social activity, or increased isolation) cannot be explained solely as a function of either the person or the environment, but, rather, explanations for behavioral change rest upon the unique confluence of biological, personality, social, situational, and cultural factors at a given time and place. Based upon the model, stability and change are viewed as a function of the complex interactions that occur between the person and environment as interdependent systems. In addition, because the person and environment are interdependent systems, change in either results in change throughout the entire system (Parmelee & Lawton, 1990).

The multiple components of the person-environment system all influence the process of change. For purposes of discussion, these multiple components can be divided into the person (both internal and external aspects) and the environment (residential and broader community). Factors internal to the person include health, mobility, attitudes and feelings, coping resources, personality, locus of control, and morale. External person factors include social resources such as income, education, socioeconomic status, marital status,

parental status, number and availability of supportive relationships, and involvement in role relationships.

The environment operates on two levels: residential and broader
community. Residential environmental factors relate to the immediate aspects of the senior housing environment. These include
physical and architectural features, social climate, aggregate staff
and tenant characteristics, and residential policies and programs.
At the other level environmental factors include the broader community, the environment in which the senior housing exists. These
broader environmental factors include geographic location, formal services available in the community, familial and other relationships outside the complex, and sociocultural events and trends.

Figure 1.1 describes the key features of the transactional model
to understand the key factors in senior housing. For professionals
working with frail elderly it is essential to understand how the
dimensions of the person and environment are interrelated. To
achieve this understanding they need specific knowledge concerning aging and aging-related changes (health, functional impairment, psychological change, role change, support systems);
knowledge of management policies and procedures; and a clear
understanding of environmental theory related to stability and
change.

Efforts to interpret and understand what is actually taking place
in senior housing require a model that is sufficiently complex to
incorporate the many diverse elements operating in senior housing that influence the processes of change. The transactional model
is useful because it helps to integrate the variety of information
that describes what is going on in senior housing and to understand the interdependence that exists between the person and
environment. The transactional model goes beyond other models
that focus solely on how the environment affects the person or the
person affects the environment. This model focuses on the changing relations between the person and environment in transaction.
For practitioners working with elderly persons with disabilities,
understanding that the person and environment are two interdependent systems provides a more realistic notion of causality
than a simple stimulus-response approach.

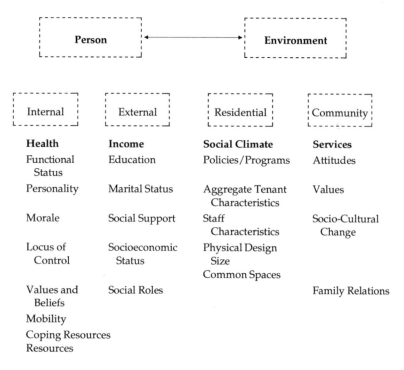

Figure 1.1. Person-Environment Transactional Model

CONCLUSION

The tremendous growth in the numbers and percentage of vulnerable elderly tenants in senior housing challenges those who work with older persons to identify successful strategies to assist at risk tenants to maintain their independence and self-determination, while at the same time to preserve the overall quality of life for all elderly tenants in senior housing. The ability to meet the challenges ahead requires building partnerships among housing managers, social service professionals, and health care providers serving older tenants. The ultimate goal of these partnerships is to enhance the quality of life of elderly tenants while preserving the dignity and self-determination of even the most functionally impaired elderly tenants.

Success in accomplishing this goal depends upon the knowledge, sensitivity, commitment, and dedication of professionals serving the elderly. Critical components of the essential knowledge base for successful work with elderly tenants are addressed in this book. These include: (a) understanding of the complex issues and changes that are summarily defined as aging in place, (b) knowledge concerning the relationship between aging and housing management issues, and (c) sensitivity to understanding the complex transactions that occur between older persons and their environment.

2

Significant Trends Affecting Senior Housing

DURING the past 30 years several major trends have raised expectations that senior housing should be more than just a place to live. The trends that have most directly influenced our thinking about senior housing are: (a) the demographic or "aging" revolution; (b) federal, state, and local housing policy initiatives concerning support services to vulnerable elderly tenants; and (c) changes in the locus of the long-term care delivery system.

THE DEMOGRAPHIC "AGING" REVOLUTION

The demographic revolution occurring in our society, popularly called the "graying of America," has had a profound impact on all aspects of American life. Today 1 out of every 9 Americans is 60 years of age and older. By 2030, 25% of the population (or one in every four Americans) will be 60 years or older. During the next 25 years the population over 60 will more than double. Increases in life expectancy due to advances in medical and health care and declines in mortality at extreme old age have significantly increased the numbers of persons who survive to old age. In 1900 there were approximately 3.1 million persons 65 years of age and older, representing 4% of the population. By 1985 the number of older persons had swelled to 29.1 million, approximately 12% of the population. By the year 2020, estimates predict the number to have increased to 54.5 million, representing about 18% of the population. Estimates predict that between 1985 and 2020 the rate of growth for the 65 and older population will be approximately 2% per year. The net result of this rate of growth is, according to Social Security Administration estimates, approximately 750,000 additional older persons every year.

Gerontologists have coined the term "aging revolution" to describe these changes because of their significant and far-reaching consequences for all the institutions within our society. As a society, however, we are only now beginning to realize the consequences of these changes for the family, the health care delivery system, the economic and political systems, social service programs, housing programs, and religious institutions.

Of all the aging demographic changes the most dramatic is the rapid rate of growth of the oldest old (85 years and older)—the fastest growing segment of our society. While today 1 out of 15 persons is 85 years of age and older, by 2030, 1 in 10 persons will be 85 and older. Between 1985 and 2020 this age group is projected to double from 1.2% to 2.4% of the population (Fisk, 1988), with estimates suggesting that by 2050 the oldest old will represent 5.2% of the population (National Institute on Aging, 1986).

The rate of growth of the oldest old raises major concerns regarding how our society will be able to respond to their needs. Because the incidence of chronic health problems and functional impairment increases with age, particularly after age 75, one major consequence of the aging revolution will be significant increases in the numbers of older persons who must rely on others to be able to carry out their essential activities of daily living. For example, estimates note that approximately one third of all persons 65 years of age and older experience some difficulty with one or more activities of daily living (e.g., bathing, dressing, shopping, housekeeping, etc.), while approximately 10% have difficulties with three or more activities of daily living. Among the oldest old, more than 60% experience difficulties with one or more activities of daily living, while about 25% had difficulty with three or more activities (National Center for Health Statistics, 1986).

As the level of functional impairment increases, the need for long-term care services also grows. For persons 65 to 74 years of age, fewer than one in seven require long-term services. Among the oldest old, however, two out of three persons need some type of long-term care services (Manton, 1984). Of those requiring long-term care services, there is a far greater need for community-based services than nursing home services. Among the oldest old approximately 46% need community-based or home-based long-term care services. In contrast, about 16% require institutionally based long-term care. (U.S. Senate, Special Committee on Aging, 1984).

Aging in place in senior housing provides concrete evidence of both the existence and consequences of the aging revolution. As tenants in elderly housing survive well into their 80s and 90s, growing numbers of tenants experience increased difficulties in being able to carry out their normal activities. Housing managers and social service and health professionals can testify to the consequences of the aging revolution because the scope and the magnitude of the problems they confront on a daily basis have increased dramatically. More and more elderly tenants/clients experience increasingly difficult, complex problems associated with advanced old age. As a result, growing numbers of managers of senior housing find that the majority of their tenants must increasingly depend on others to carry out their essential activities of daily living. As levels of frailty increase, the challenge for housing managers, social service providers, and health care professionals is to devise innovative support systems and approaches that enable at risk or impaired elderly tenants to live independently in the community.

FEDERAL, STATE, AND LOCAL INITIATIVES
TO PROVIDE SERVICES IN SENIOR HOUSING

A second trend that has influenced our thinking about senior housing is an assortment of demonstration projects and special initiatives conducted during the past 30 years that have sought to introduce supportive services into senior housing. Increased expectations about the need for supportive services in traditional senior housing can be linked to repeated attempts to test the feasibility of supportive services in independent age-segregated housing. While no one supportive services initiative can be directly linked to the development of either permanent comprehensive mechanisms for services or direct service subsidies, the cumulative impact of these demonstration projects has been to increase expectations that senior housing should provide support to elderly tenants. The following brief survey of developments in the field of housing highlights how these demonstration projects and supportive service initiatives have raised expectations about services.

The Federal Response

The federal government has been reluctant to formulate specific policies concerning the need for supportive services in senior housing (Harel & Harel, 1978; Lawton, Moss, & Grimes, 1985; Sheehan, 1987). As early as the 1960s, however, there were a limited number of federally sponsored housing initiatives addressing the support needs of elderly tenants (Sheehan, 1987). The earliest evidence of the federal government's response to meeting the support needs of tenants comes from several small-scale demonstration projects designed to provide services to vulnerable or impaired elderly tenants (Bevis & Bing, 1961).

One federal initiative related to expectations for supportive services in senior housing, the Housing Act of 1970, authorized support for the construction of service spaces such as dining rooms and kitchens. No operating subsidies were provided, however, to cover the cost of the purchase, preparation, or serving of meals. Subsequent legislation, the Housing and Community Development Act of 1974, specified the need for services in subsidized housing but did not provide funds for operating service programs. During the past 30 years the federal government, while recognizing the need for supportive services in subsidized housing, has failed to provide operating subsidies to assure that elderly tenants with disabilities will receive needed support services.

In 1978 the Congregate Housing Services Act (CHSP) authorized limited funds on a demonstration basis to test the cost-effectiveness of supportive services in subsidized housing. This legislation enabled HUD to enter into contracts with either public housing authorities or Section 202 borrowers for services to elderly tenants with disabilities and handicapped tenants. The service package included a mandatory meal service and the provision of other services to enable individuals to remain living independently.

Initial passage of the Congregate Housing Services Act in the mid-1970s heightened expectations that the federal government would increasingly respond to the support needs of vulnerable elderly tenants, however, both the Reagan and Bush administrations have sought to eliminate the CHSP. Despite this opposition, Congress has continued to authorize the program. Appropriations for fiscal years 1989 and 1990 are $5.4 million and $5.8 million. As of 1988 there were 60 CHSP programs serving approximately 2,000 residents (U.S. Senate, Special Committee on Aging, 1990). Because the CHSP serves a small fraction of elderly tenants in need of supportive services, critics have argued that the program has diverted attention from the need for a more comprehensive program that meets the support needs of the vast majority of vulnerable senior housing tenants who live in complexes not served by the CHSP. The underlying philosophy of the program, however, reinforced expectations that vulnerable senior housing tenants should be maintained in their housing complexes with support services.

For proponents who favor a strong federal role in housing, the 1980s have been a very disappointing period. Since 1981 the federal involvement in housing has been radically reduced due primarily to a major shift in the philosophy of both the Reagan and Bush administrations toward the federal government's role in housing. Major reductions in HUD appropriations during the 1980s significantly limited the production of housing units. HUD appropriations for assisted housing dropped from $25 billion in 1981 to $8.9 billion in 1990, representing a reduction of more than 80% when inflation is computed in (U.S. Senate, Special Committee on Aging, 1990).

Despite this bleak picture, federal legislation offers some hope that there will be a renewed response on the part of the federal government in the 1990s. The Cranston-Gonzales National Affordable Housing Act, to a limited extent, addresses the supportive service needs of older persons residing in federally assisted housing. A component of this bill calls for an Assistant Secretary for Supportive Housing with responsibility for overseeing housing programs serving the elderly, handicapped, and homeless. Included under the provisions of this bill is a new title—Housing for Persons with Special Needs—to assure that elderly housing will be designed to meet the needs of all persons with disabilities and to upgrade existing elderly housing. Additional features of the bill include the provision of salaries for supportive services coordinators in public housing and funding for supportive services in cooperation with state and local partnerships. The legislation provides an incentive for the provision of services to elderly tenants with disabilities.

State and Local Supportive Services Initiatives

During the 1980s, as the federal government diminished its role in housing and supportive services, the importance of state and local responses increased. State-sponsored congregate services programs vary widely from state to state with respect to the type and frequency of support services, the service subsidy, the mix of frail to independent tenants, and the method of service delivery.

Senior housing complexes have attempted to secure support services for at risk elderly tenants on the local level. These efforts have resulted in a wide variety of services in senior housing. These include: transportation, meals, senior center activities, visiting nurse services, and social and recreation programs. These community services, however, lack coordination and fail to serve the needs of the most impaired tenants. This approach to services has been termed the "patchwork" approach because it depends on piecing together existing community services (Lawton et al., 1985). There are a number of problems, however, with this approach. For instance, a needed service may not be available in the local community. Furthermore, the reliability of the patchwork of services in assuring that older tenants' needs are met depends on continued appropriations for community-based services at sufficient levels to meet tenants' needs. With continued cutbacks in human services programs, the feasibility of the patchwork approach for meeting the support needs of tenants must be seriously questioned.

The fiscal restraints that limit the availability of community-based services are a major obstacle to assuring the needs of elderly tenants with disabilities will be met. Further, housing management's reliance on services from community agencies puts them in a "begging" position to secure the needed services (Christensen & Cranz, 1987). Given the limited appropriations for community services, there are too few services to meet the needs of elderly tenants and other groups of community-living elderly persons. Another problem associated with the patchwork approach to services is the inexperience of most housing managers in managing or securing services. Finally, when services are provided by a variety of different local community service agencies, there is a lack of communication among the different service providers. Housing managers frequently complain about the lack of communication among the community agencies providing the services and the exclusion of housing staff from decision making concerning elderly tenants.

In briefly highlighting some of the major program initiatives that have impacted on the senior housing industry—the CHSP, state congregate services programs, and local service initiatives— there seems little doubt that senior housing complexes are increasingly expected to identify ways to respond to the support needs of elderly tenants.

CHANGES IN THE LOCUS OF THE LONG-TERM CARE DELIVERY SYSTEM

A third influence that has increased expectations for services in senior housing is a gradual shift in the locus of the long-term care delivery system from institutional care to community-based care. As a result, various types of planned housing are increasingly defined as part of the long-term care continuum. Congregate housing, board and care homes, continuing care retirement communities, and even traditional senior housing have all been mentioned as part of the long-term care continuum serving the needs of elderly persons. The movement to serve older persons in the least restrictive environment has created pressures on housing managers to maintain at risk older persons in their own homes.

Given the tremendous differences that exist in the availability of support services both among and within these different categories of specialized housing, however, great caution is deemed necessary before such conclusions are warranted, particularly for traditional senior housing, because few housing complexes provide a range of supportive services sufficient to assist functionally impaired elderly tenants.

Due to increased efforts to contain the excessive costs of institutional care and reduce unnecessary institutional placements in long-term care facilities, managers of senior housing find themselves responsible for managing increasingly impaired, functionally dependent elderly tenants who suffer multiple chronic health problems, but who are judged inappropriate for nursing home placement.

Although senior housing is increasingly viewed as part of the long-term care continuum, there is no systematic public policy that links together housing, health, social service, welfare, and income maintenance to serve the needs of elderly tenants with disabilities (Tilson & Fahey, 1990). The lack of systematic public policies and operating subsidies creates major problems for housing managers and social service providers who seek to maintain functionally impaired elderly tenants in the community. The lack of a comprehensive policy results in the inability to deliver the critical components of the long-term care system to elderly tenants—coordination, monitoring, and assessment. Instead, the services elderly tenants receive are characterized by fragmentation among the diverse components of the long-term care delivery system. While community-based services, such as home care, Meals on Wheels, adult day care programs, chore services, have become an increased presence in the day-to-day management of senior housing, there are no provisions within senior housing that enable the overall monitoring or coordination of these services.

As a result of pressures to maintain increasingly dependent, functionally impaired tenants in the community, housing managers struggle to determine when a tenant is no longer appropriate for the particular housing environment. With these increased pressures, assessment has become a critical component of the management function. Few managers, however, have adequate knowledge of assessment strategies or tools.

CONCLUSION

Overall the impact of the demographic revolution, the service demonstration projects, and the changing locus of the long-term care system have dramatically altered senior housing. Not only are elderly tenants living in senior housing to advanced old age, but also more and more elderly tenants are experiencing increased levels of frailty. As a result, housing managers and social service and health professionals are dealing with growing numbers of vulnerable or at risk elderly tenants who need support. As the numbers and percentage of elderly tenants with disabilities in senior housing have increased, so have expectations that support- ive services to assist elderly tenants should be incorporated into senior housing. Because the overwhelming majority of senior housing complexes operate without any service subsidy, how- ever, housing managers are left to formulate their own policies regarding how to respond to the "aging" of their tenants.

In looking to the future, the development of a comprehensive policy that links together housing, health care, and social services is critically needed. There are multiple barriers that create prob- lems in achieving this goal however (Pynoos, 1990). Barriers that prevent passage of legislation to enable the provision of services in independent senior housing include: (a) political fragmentation and territoriality concerning the domains of health, housing, and social services, which fails to bring together these different groups; (b) program inflexibility concerning benefits, reimbursement, and staffing; (c) Reaganomics; and (d) the federal deficit.

At the federal level the recent signing of memoranda of under- standing between the Administration on Aging and the Depart- ment of Housing and Urban Development and Farmers Home Administration offers some promise that there is movement, how- ever limited, toward integrating supportive services into senior housing.

3

The Changing Role of Housing Manager: Redefining the Role and Responsibilities of Housing Managers

Elderly tenants frequently turn to housing managers to handle their personal problems, provide emotional support and counseling, resolve disputes with other tenants, make sense out of medical bills and paperwork, and provide a helping hand or ready ear to listen to tenants' concerns.

THE increased attention focused on the role of senior housing in meeting the needs of elderly residents raises numerous questions concerning the role and responsibilities of housing managers in senior housing. This chapter addresses the following questions:

1. Who are the managers in senior housing?
2. How has the role of housing manager changed over the past 20 years?

3. What are the appropriate roles and responsibilities of senior housing managers?
4. How do views of "autonomy" impact on how elderly tenants are treated?

WHO ARE HOUSING MANAGERS IN SENIOR HOUSING?

If you were to gather together 100 housing managers, there would be 100 different stories about how each person became a housing manager. A few examples illustrate the point that housing managers are a diverse group. Informal conversations with housing managers at a recent training workshop identified ministers, former housewives, several former tenants, and an unemployed engineer, all who had found their way to become managers in elderly housing. Most had been in the field 10 years or more, while a few had recently become housing managers. Few had any specific training in housing management prior to their first job and none had any formal training in gerontology.

What is clear is that persons who manage senior housing complexes are an extremely heterogeneous group. The diversity is seen with respect to their background characteristics (age, sex, years of formal education, prior training and experience, etc.), past and present administrative responsibilities (e.g., number of units, size of staff, management style, etc.), overall experience in elderly housing (number of years in the field), and personal qualities (interpersonal skills, acceptance of older persons, sensitivity to aging issues, ability to handle stress, acceptance of own aging, etc.).

All, however, must deal with aging-related physical, social, and psychological problems that challenge the most well-trained gerontologists: incontinence, paranoia, depression, suicide, grief, functional impairment, caregiver stress and burden, Alzheimer's disease, sensory impairment, falls and broken hips, wandering, and so on.

A typical day in a housing manager's life includes dealing with tenants' complaints about a wandering tenant, contacting a family to try to convince them that their elderly relative requires a more supportive housing environment due to increasing cognitive impairment, responding to an emergency call when a tenant falls in her bathroom, arranging for the ambulance, interviewing prospective tenants for the complex, meetings with several tenants who have complaints about a tenant's incontinence, collecting rents, and attending the monthly tenant meeting. Housing managers increasingly find themselves performing many different activities that are subsumed under their role. Formal job descriptions for housing managers, however, fail to reflect the full range of these everyday activities.

The gap between what housing managers actually do and formal job descriptions creates a good deal of confusion when attempting to define their actual responsibilities. In part, this confusion stems from the failure of housing sponsors to incorporate new responsibilities into the formal definition of the job. Viewed from a role theory perspective, there are advantages and disadvantages associated with the lack of explicit job responsibilities. On the one hand, the lack of clear cut expectations associated with the role of housing manager leaves individual housing managers with some freedom in how they define their role. A recent national survey of housing managers of section 202 housing confirms the existence of wide individual differences in the way housing managers define the job and allocate their time (U.S. House of Representatives Select Committee on Aging, 1989). While the lack of specific job performance criteria enables housing managers some latitude in the way they allocate their time, on the other hand, poorly defined role expectations create ambiguity concerning rewards for "good" job performance. Recent efforts to help housing managers redefine their role to include expanded functions, such as care managers, have generally not addressed the need to incorporate these new responsibilities into more formal job descriptions. The following sections discuss the emerging role of the housing manager and the key components associated with this new role.

MANAGING SENIOR HOUSING: A UNIQUE MANAGEMENT ROLE

In the past the role of senior housing manager was primarily defined as that of landlord or property manager. Trained as landlords, they had administrative responsibility for collecting rents; renting out vacant units; overseeing lease and contractual compliance; overseeing the maintenance of the buildings and grounds; supervising staff; preparing operating budgets; completing regulatory paperwork; developing residential policies and procedures; screening prospective tenants; handling complaints from tenants, families, and staff; and responding to all emergencies (Pynoos, 1990).

As the demands of aging tenants in senior housing have changed, housing managers have been called upon to perform extensive tasks that go beyond their typical "landlord" responsibilities. Tasks associated with the emerging management role include provision of information and referral to elderly tenants, monitoring the supportive services that vulnerable tenants receive, and providing counseling and emotional support to elderly tenants. In addition, housing managers are expected to establish a supportive environment that enhances the well-being of elderly tenants and encourages social involvement among residents.

Few people appreciate how difficult and rewarding it is to be a manager of senior housing. While a manager has responsibility for all the administrative aspects of housing, he or she is also expected to be much more actively involved and concerned about the welfare and quality of life for all his or her elderly residents (Patterson, 1990).

As new responsibilities emerge, housing managers must successfully integrate both the administrative and support aspects of their job. In expanding their role, housing managers must establish reasonable boundaries between their responsibilities and those of other professionals serving elderly tenants. In general, far more work has focused on identifying the expanded functions that housing managers perform than in helping managers either establish boundaries concerning their role or integrate new responsibilities into their existing role.

HOUSING MANAGERS AS CARE MANAGERS

Several housing experts have recently identified housing managers as care managers (Sykes, 1989) or case managers (Hofland,

1990). The work of James Sykes, Center for Health Sciences at the University of Wisconsin-Madison, is particularly helpful in delineating the responsibilities of housing managers as care managers (Sykes, 1989). According to Sykes, housing managers should be "care managers" for those elderly tenants who have difficulty in being self-sufficient and who lack sufficient support from other sources. The responsibilities for care managers, according to Sykes (1989), are to provide "guidance, support and timely intervention" (p. 11) for tenants in need.

The role of care manager comes about because for many elderly tenants the housing manager is the primary "caring" person to whom tenants can turn in times of need. Responsibilities as care manager, however, do not replace administrative responsibilities; rather, they are added on to housing managers' many administrative tasks. Sykes (1989) provides some general guidelines for how this integration can be achieved. First, because new responsibilities as care managers are added on to administrative tasks, housing managers must constantly seek to balance their administrative and care responsibilities. Achieving this balance, however, is not an easy task. Second, housing managers as care managers must balance their time and attention in managing care to assure that the needs of all tenants are met. Third, housing managers must delegate caring responsibilities to involve others in the provision of care to frail older tenants. Without such sharing of responsibility, a manager will find there is too little time and too many needs. Given the tremendous constraints on housing managers' time and resources that impact on their ability to be care managers, Sykes has identified three strategies that housing managers should employ to effectively assume the responsibility as care managers.

Care managers should: (a) promote independence and self-determination even among the frailest residents, (b) involve others in the provision of care and assistance to elderly tenants, and (c) create a naturally caring and supportive environment.

1. As care managers, housing managers must continually work to promote independence and self-determination among even the frailest residents. To develop interventions that promote independence, care managers must accurately know each tenant's overall competence level. Needed interventions must begin at the level of the tenant and seek to increase his or her personal skills or

competencies and/or the availability of socially supportive relationships. Effective care managers do not perform all support activities for elderly tenants. Attempts to do everything for tenants promote dependence, take time away from other responsibilities, and diminish the importance of other supportive relationships in tenants' lives. Whenever appropriate, it is far more desirable for housing managers to provide information to tenants concerning community agencies that provide needed services, than for the housing manager to make the call. It is important that housing managers provide vulnerable, functionally impaired tenants with sufficient support to assure that their efforts to access services will promote feelings of self-determination and self-worth. Taking time to explain how to contact a particular agency, the kinds of responses he or she might expect, and what to do under certain circumstances prepares the tenant for handling this new encounter with a formal service agency. The tenant who has learned to access the needed service has increased his or her ability to handle future problems. In contrast, if the housing manager has made the call, the tenant has learned to handle future problems by bringing his or her problems to the housing manager when the problems arise.

2. Care managers need to involve others in providing support and assistance to elderly tenants with disabilities. It is impractical, inefficient, and counterproductive for housing managers alone to provide assistance to elderly tenants. Housing managers as care managers need to identify others to provide support to elderly tenants. This may include helping uninvolved relatives to recognize the importance of their help, developing resident "caring and sharing" committees, or encouraging naturally occurring informal assistance among tenants. "Enlisting allies" (Sykes, 1989) serves to increase the size of the support network serving at risk elderly tenants. Tenants with extremely limited support systems are particularly vulnerable during times of stress. Family, friends, clergy, health care professionals, friendly visitors, and social workers are potential allies to expand the support network of elderly tenants.

3. Housing managers should create a naturally caring and supportive environment. Housing managers have responsibility for creating an environment that encourages neighbors to care for the welfare of one another. Housing managers, however, need to be

sensitive to helping aging tenants set realistic expectations for themselves about helping. Housing managers should help tenants understand the value of the different types of support they can provide to one another. Help is frequently defined as assistance with instrumental activities, such as shopping, cleaning, and meal preparation (Sheehan, 1988b). Yet this is only one aspect of support or assistance. Housing managers need to be sensitive to the strong psychological feelings that emerge in unbalanced helping relationships and to seek ways of promoting a supportive environment that minimizes the costs for both functionally impaired elderly tenants and independent tenants. On the one hand, efforts should be made to identify ways to enable vulnerable tenants to maintain their sense of autonomy, while on the other hand, the healthier, more independent tenants must be assisted in defining appropriate ways of supporting elderly tenants with disabilities.

Although housing managers have no formal responsibility for care management, these functions inevitably arise as part of the management role. Providing residents with information about community services and programs, counseling tenants, making decisions concerning whether elderly tenants can remain in the housing environment, and ensuring that elderly tenants are receiving necessary supportive services to avoid future crises are all components of the care manager role. According to Brian Hofland (1990), "The question is not whether managers should take on a case management role, but how they can improve their performance in that role or delegate aspects of it to other appropriately trained professionals" (p. 254).

CONCERNS ABOUT HOUSING MANAGERS AS CARE MANAGERS

While there is growing acceptance of the emerging role of housing manager as care manager, several concerns are associated with the emergence of this new role. First, as housing managers take on the added responsibilities, they must constantly work to balance the multiple demands on their time and attention. The balancing requires achieving equilibrium between the demands of administrative responsibilities and tenant services responsibilities. What is unclear for housing managers is how this balance should be achieved. Does equilibrium between administration and tenant services mean roughly dividing the hours worked between these two major responsibilities? Further, because as senior housing complexes "age", tenants' needs for services increase, how should housing managers adjust the balance between administrative responsibilities and tenant service needs over time?

A second concern associated with the expanded view of the role of housing manager is the stress associated with the increased demands on housing managers. Housing managers who attempt to act as care managers, but are unable to meet the competing demands on their time, will experience excessive stress that can lead to burnout. Unless housing managers are able to develop effective coping strategies and intervention strategies for working with elderly tenants with disabilities, burnout is inevitable.

Third, the expanded view of housing managers as care managers may be misinterpreted. Housing managers who equate this new role with "taking care of elderly tenants" may become overly protective of elderly tenants. Overly helpful or protective housing managers, however, deprive elderly tenants of their rights for self-determination and independence. Housing managers should be constantly aware that, as Lawton (1975) states, "it is a very short distance from the wish to help to the compulsion to dominate" (p. 231).

Finally, the tasks associated with the care manager role presuppose a knowledge about aging, interpersonal relations, personal counseling skills, assessment, and community services that many housing managers lack. If the new role of care manager is to be effectively implemented, concerted efforts must be directed at educating housing managers about these complex issues and methods of intervention that promote the quality of life of older persons.

GUIDELINES FOR CARE MANAGERS
WORKING WITH ELDERLY TENANTS

James Sykes (1989) provides helpful guidelines for care managers to enhance elderly tenants' well-being and self-esteem and to protect the care manager from excess stress and burnout:

1. Protect the resident's dignity at all costs. Always treat residents as adults. Anticipate their needs so they need not continually ask for help. Older people have a right to be involved in decisions affecting them, and, whenever possible, reverse the roles: ask for resident's help rather than always offering yours.

2. Recognize that underneath some expressions of independence is a real but silent need. Out of a deep-seated sense of rugged individualism and years of overcoming hardship, older people want to be seen as independent even when reality dictates otherwise. As you work with people who may need to enter a nursing home, remember to sort out claims of independence from facts about their needs. By doing so, and by anticipating problems, you can help residents become more accepting of their circumstances. That can make a necessary move far less threatening.

3. Guard against any erosion of a resident's right to decide. Often out of a well-motivated desire to do what is right for a frail resident, managers and family members make plans without consulting the resident. While such concern shows caring and a sense of responsibility, plans made without the resident's full involvement violate a precious right of self-determination.

4. Separate your well-being from that of residents. It is difficult to approach a resident's problem without seeing it from your own perspective. Walking in another's shoes is impossible, yet it is vital to try, especially when a decision affects not only a resident but also the image of your residence. The extent to which you keep residents' interests at the center of your daily responsibilities determines the success of your housing—for both manager and residents.

5. Be a friend first and then a manager. A friend keeps other's needs clearly in mind and brings a great deal of caring to a friendship. Friends like being together, and while it is impossible for a manager to spend hours and hours being a friend, it is important that a personal relationship develop between manager and resident so both may feel their place is like a home, not an institution.

6. Take care of yourself, too. In any caring enterprise it is all too easy for the problems of others to overwhelm the feelings of professionals on the scene. Spending time alone with a spouse or colleague who faces similar challenges is vital to the mental health of every professional, especially those who help others through difficult times. Otherwise you may find your reservoir of good will and judgment registering "empty." Of course you must be ready whenever a crisis arises, but take time to discover the balance between caring for others and caring for yourself. (pp. 20-21)

SOURCE: Sykes (1989). Reprinted with permission.

OTHER ROLES FOR HOUSING MANAGERS

Other roles for housing managers either subsumed under the care manager role or enacted alone emerge from the expanded view of senior housing. These roles include: empowerer, advocate, coordinator, facilitator, developer, linker, and resource person (Biegel, Shore, & Gordon, 1984). The underlying rationale for these new roles is the need to overcome the many barriers that prevent the full mobilization of the support system serving elderly tenants and to reduce the gaps and fragmentation in the service delivery system. While there is some overlap among these different activities/functions, each activity is oriented toward a different goal.

Empowerer

Housing managers empower elderly tenants when they encourage, support, and facilitate elderly tenants' rights for personal control and self-determination. Actions that empower elderly tenants include: (a) implementation of residential policies and structures that maximize tenant involvement in decision making, (b) provision of information concerning existing community services and entitlement programs, (c) reinforcement of positive social interaction and social skills, (d) respect for the dignity and the privacy of the individual, and (e) provision of educational and personal growth programs for elderly tenants.

Advocate

Housing managers serve as advocates for elderly tenants when they assist them in obtaining needed services and resources. Advocacy efforts may include: (a) bringing community services on-site to better serve tenants, (b) encouraging formal and quasi-formal support organizations to develop needed services, (c) working on community councils on aging to represent the needs of elderly tenants, and (d) networking with social service and health professionals to assure that tenants receive the services that they need.

Coordinator

Given the fragmentation of the formal support system, housing managers can direct their efforts to bring together existing services to provide a more comprehensive base of services that elderly tenants receive. Working with social service providers, health care professionals, and community service organizations, managers can attempt to bring a comprehensive package of support services into the housing complex to meet the needs of elderly tenants.

Facilitator

The overall purpose of this role is to enable elderly tenants to receive needed services and entitlements. A variety of activities are part of the facilitator role. Any activity that reduces barriers that prevent older persons from receiving needed services is included under this role. Examples of activities include: (a) offering informational programs regarding community services or entitlement programs, (b) assistance with paper work, (c) help in dealing with the bureaucracy, and (d) sponsorship of activities or programs for family members.

Initiator/Developer

Housing managers who identify an unmet need among elderly tenants can develop innovative service programs to meet tenant need. Examples of innovative service programs serving frail elderly tenants in senior housing are discussed in Chapter 8, "Formal Services in Senior Housing."

Linker: Intrasystem

Housing managers who assume this role work to strengthen the support tenants receive from family, friends, and neighbors. Chapter 7, "Social Support in the Lives of Elderly Tenants" provides suggestions for facilitating support within the informal support system for meeting the needs of elderly tenants.

Linker: Intersystem

This role involves activities designed to coordinate services provided by the formal and informal support systems to better serve the needs of frail elderly tenants. Because multiple barriers (e.g., lack of knowledge, fear of formal services, personal and family values) prevent elderly tenants and their families from accessing needed services, housing managers may work to reduce or eliminate these barriers.

Resource Provider

An essential activity of housing managers is the provision of resources (information) to elderly tenants and members of their informal support system to assure that their support needs are met.

The new roles for housing managers are clearly not mutually exclusive. Housing managers may take on one or all of these new roles. In determining the appropriateness or relevance of each role, housing managers need to assess both tenant need and their own personal skills and competence to enact the role.

PROMOTING AUTONOMY
AMONG ELDERLY TENANTS

An overriding issue concerning the enactment of the role of housing manager is how housing managers promote autonomy and independence among elderly tenants. Whether functioning as a more traditional housing manager or a care manager, the overall goals of housing management should focus on ways of promoting the autonomy and dignity of the individual. The housing manager's conception of "autonomy" directly influences his or her interactions with elderly tenants (Hofland, 1990). Different actions toward elderly tenants on the part of housing managers, in part, reflect differing philosophical views of autonomy. These different views or conceptions have been labeled "negative" and "positive" autonomy (Hofland, 1990). On the one hand, housing managers who maintain a negative view of autonomy assume that autonomy is achieved through noninterference in the lives of elderly tenants. Tenants are "left alone" so that they exercise control over their lives. On the other hand, housing managers who maintain a positive view of autonomy believe in the importance of providing resources that promote resident autonomy.

These different conceptions of autonomy have obvious implications for how the housing manager role is enacted. According to Hofland (1990):

> The manager who holds a notion of negative autonomy essentially says,
> "I respect the autonomy of this resident so much that I will leave her alone so that she is free to make any decision that she chooses as long as she doesn't violate her housing contract. She is an adult and doesn't need any meddling from me in any way."
> The manager who holds a positive notion of autonomy says, "I respect the autonomy of this resident so much that I will do everything within my ability to empower and support her in fulfilling her potential within this setting so that she can be as autonomous as possible." (p. 261)

Housing managers and social service providers should take time to think about their personal conception of autonomy and repertoire of strategies that they use to promote positive autonomy. Clearly all intervention strategies that housing managers employ do not promote autonomy. Interventions aimed at empowering tenants and/or increasing their potential to cope with future problems are aimed at promoting positive autonomy. Conceptions of positive autonomy should underlie all interactions with elderly tenants, even the most vulnerable tenants.

BOUNDARIES: THE DIMENSIONS OF THE HOUSING MANAGER ROLE

Finally, any discussion of the expanded role of housing manager should include mention of the boundaries of this expanded role. As new responsibilities are added, the question arises, How does the scope of this new role differ from that of social workers, case managers, and counselors? Boundaries in defining the new role of housing manager are necessary to assist housing managers in identifying the necessary and appropriate response when problems arise. Boundaries also help to set realistic limits concerning what the housing manager can and cannot accomplish given his or her knowledge and skills.

Regrettably very limited attention has been directed at helping housing managers to define the boundaries of their role. Our own work in this area has made us aware how difficult it is to resolve the issue of boundaries (Philbrick, Sheehan, & Blank, 1991; Sheehan, 1991). Interactions with a wide range of housing managers suggest that there is little consensus among housing managers regarding the boundaries that circumscribe their role. At one extreme are housing managers who define their role solely as property management, while at the other extreme are managers who do not distinguish between the normal day-to-day tasks they perform and those performed by social workers or trained counselors. For housing managers, the failure or inability to establish clear boundaries concerning the limits of their role will eventually result in role overload and confusion. Doing too much or doing it all is counterproductive for the elderly tenants, the housing manager, and opportunities to work together with trained professionals in the community who serve older adults. Further, interventions by housing managers that go beyond their training and ability can lead to serious negative consequences for the elderly tenant.

As housing managers redefine their role in meeting the needs of frail elderly tenants, they should realistically assess their knowledge and ability to take on certain roles, their ability to delegate responsibility for elderly tenants, and their knowledge of community service providers available to provide needed services. In attempting to meet the needs of elderly tenants with disabilities, housing managers should build partnerships with social service and health professionals to effectively meet tenants' needs. The manager of senior housing is successful when he or she works with social service and health professionals to meet the needs of all elderly tenants.

CONCLUSION

As the role of housing manager in senior housing has changed, there is a need to carefully consider the consequences of these changes for housing managers and the elderly tenants whom they serve. Housing managers in their efforts to meet the needs of increasing numbers of elderly tenants must constantly struggle to achieve a reasonable balance between their administrative and caring responsibilities. This is not always an easy task. Housing managers should guard against becoming involved in complex problems that go beyond their training and expertise.

Housing managers should always remember that successful management depends upon: (a) respect for the autonomy and self-determination of individual tenants, (b) delegation of responsibility, (c) knowledge about aging and aging-related problems, (d) provision of useful information and referral services, and (e) caring.

4

Management Practices and Policies and Aging in Place

SUCCESSFUL management in elderly housing creates a safe, pleasant, and secure environment that betters the quality of life for all elderly tenants. In contrast, poor, ineffective, and incompetent management increases problems, contributes to resident dissatisfaction and turmoil, and diminishes the quality of life for elderly residents (Butterfield & Weidemann, 1987). This chapter examines selected management practices and residential policies in senior housing. It also addresses the role of assessment as part of the management process.

DIMENSIONS OF MANAGEMENT IN SENIOR HOUSING

Essential management functions in senior housing are divided into three broad categories: physical, social, and financial (Patterson, 1990). While these management tasks are part of the operation of any housing facility, they take on special importance in managing senior housing. In senior housing the housing manager and staff must be continually active and vigilant to assure that the housing meets the needs of aging tenants (Patterson, 1990).

Management of the Physical Plant

Management of the physical plant is especially important in senior housing because it can: (a) create a warm, cheerful environment; (b) enhance a sense of pride and well-being among elderly tenants; and (c) reduce injuries and accidents (Patterson, 1990).

Proper maintenance of the physical plant and upkeep of the grounds are important for tenants' psychological well-being. Like people of any age, elderly tenants who live in attractive, clean, and well-maintained housing are more likely to feel a sense of pride and attachment to home than those who live in drab, unattractive, and poorly maintained buildings. For elderly tenants, living in unattractive, poorly maintained housing promotes feelings of alienation and deprivation. For tenants who are homebound, the importance of their surroundings increases as their "world" becomes defined by the confines of the complex and their own apartment. (Chapter 5 discusses the importance of design and the physical environment in promoting the well-being of elderly tenants.)

Through proper maintenance of facilities, housing managers can significantly reduce the "costs" incurred when elderly tenants suffer serious accidents. While it is impossible to calculate the exact "savings" achieved, proper maintenance can reduce the personal, psychological, social, and health care costs that occur when elderly tenants suffer serious falls or accidents.

The experiences of Mrs. H, age 79, who has lived in elderly housing for the past 9 years, provide dramatic evidence of the "costs" incurred when a serious accident occurs.

Mrs. H was always one of the most socially active tenants until last winter when she fell and broke her hip. Her fall was caused by a large, deep crack in the cement sidewalk outside of her apartment. Although she has physically recovered from her broken hip, Mrs. H has developed a "fear of falling" that prevents her from resuming her previous levels of social activity. Her progressive social isolation has led to feelings of loneliness and depression. As indicated more in detail in Chapter 5, through monitoring the physical plant, potentially dangerous aspects of the physical environment that lead to serious accidents can be eliminated.

Management of the Social Environment

Housing managers are responsible for creating a socially supportive environment for all tenants. To accomplish this goal, they must identify ways to promote a positive social climate and to provide meaningful activities for tenants. Given the importance of the social environment in senior housing, Chapter 6 provides an in-depth look at the dimensions of the social environment.

Creation of a positive social climate should focus on ways of facilitating both formal and informal social participation among elderly tenants. Formal social and educational programs are an important part of the social environment. Formal programs provide opportunities for tenants to get to know others, receive information on topics such as health and health promotion, nutrition, exercise, and current events, and offer opportunities for personal growth. Bringing community groups into the housing facility helps to reduce barriers between older tenants and the broader community.

Housing managers should encourage activities that enhance opportunities for tenants to exercise control over their environment. Examples include tenant councils, social and educational programming committees, caring and sharing committees, and newcomers committees.

From a prospective tenant's first encounter with the housing manager and throughout the tenant's tenure in the housing, the housing manager should provide a role model for friendliness, kindness, trustworthiness, and respect for individuals' dignity and privacy.

Financial Management

Proper financial management is a prerequisite for assuring adequate maintenance of the physical plant and promoting elderly tenants' sense of security in being able to afford to live in their home (Patterson, 1990). Because most elderly tenants are on a fixed income, long-range budgets must accurately anticipate funds to cover normal maintenance of the physical facility and unexpected repairs that will inevitably occur. Adequate long-range financial planning should guard against the necessity of dramatic increases in rent, which tenants on a fixed income cannot easily absorb. Large unanticipated rent increases can cause tenants to feel alienated and distrustful of the management and insecure about future rent increases.

Because all three dimensions of management—physical, social, financial—are interrelated, successful managers must perform all three functions. If the manager assumes responsibility for only one or two functions, attempts to provide a supportive, satisfying environment for elderly tenants will be unsuccessful (Patterson, 1990).

Residential Policies: A Key Factor in Successful Management

As growing numbers of elderly tenants experience limitations in their ability to care for themselves and live independently, the importance of clear-cut residential policies has increased dramatically. Well-formulated residential policies help housing managers to:

- Achieve long-range goals
- Enhance communication between management and residents
- Protect the rights of residents
- Ensure tenants' right to appeal decisions
- Protect the housing manager and staff from liability
- Facilitate decision making

Residential policies are a means of achieving the long-range goals of the housing complex and of anticipating the future needs of elderly tenants. Although many of the changes that occur in senior housing are beyond the control of the housing manager, careful attention to residential policies provides mechanisms to proactively respond to the challenges of aging in place. In the long run, decisions that enable extremely frail tenants to remain in senior housing must be associated with increased efforts to secure supportive services (Lawton, Greenbaum, & Liebowitz, 1980). Housing managers should consider how their screening, admission, retention, and discharge policies impact both the housing environment and the aggregate characteristics of the tenant population. Retention policies that enable frail or marginal tenants to remain in the housing complex create an aggregate profile of predominately frail, impaired tenants. Over time the "image" of the housing complex will be that of an older more functionally impaired population, and this will affect the characteristics of later applicants (Lawton et al., 1980).

Developing Residential Policies

Essential policies should provide tenants with information concerning the nature of the housing complex, their rights and responsibilities, and their right to appeal decisions.

Policies can also serve to protect the housing manager and staff from liability and assist them in decision making when a tenant can no longer live in independent housing. Within the limits of federal, state, and local statutes regarding fair housing and civil rights, housing managers should consider the importance of clear and consistent residential policies and procedures for guiding the operation of their housing.

A recent court case involving a 90-year-old woman who was transferred from her senior housing apartment to a nursing home illustrates the "costliness" of poorly developed residential policies.

A 90-year-old resident in a senior housing facility sued the housing staff and the Department of Social Services after being transferred to a nursing home. The woman's lawyer argued that "neither the highrise nor the Department of Social Services provided the resident or her family with adequate communication regarding the transfer and violated her rights in moving her to a nursing home"

The case was decided in favor of the plaintiff, who was awarded a "sizeable sum." The decision against the housing staff and Department of Social Services focused on the need for clear communication and the protection of the tenant's rights. (Hellman, 1990, p. 101).

The following guidelines identify some of the key elements that should be included in the development of residential policies. According to Hellman (1990), policies in senior housing should specify:

- Who makes decisions
- What are the circumstances that require relocation to supportive housing
- Procedures for assessing all tenants
- Specific procedures for communicating with elderly tenants
- Mechanisms for making tenants aware of their rights to appeal

In reviewing their residential policies, housing managers need to consider whether their screening, admission, and relocation policies meet the criteria for effective housing policy.

Screening. Screening is a management process for assuring that applicants to the housing complex demonstrate the capacity to meet the conditions under the lease. Failure to adequately screen prospective tenants impacts both the financial solvency of the complex and the quality of life for all tenants. Screening policies provide guidelines for housing managers to determine whether an applicant to the housing will be able to meet the requirements under the lease. Screening cannot and should not be used to exclude prospective tenants arbitrarily. Owners and housing managers may not discriminate based upon race, color, creed, religion, sex, national origin, age, or handicap. Screening assessments should focus exclusively on the individual's capacity to perform tasks related to his or her competence in being able to meet the conditions of the lease.

A memorandum from the U.S. Office of Housing and Urban Development Region I Office (1991) underscores the importance of screening for the successful operation of subsidized housing. It reads:

While owners are responsible to assure that subsidized residents meet eligibility criteria for subsidy, this does not mean that owners must accept into residency anybody who meets the eligibility criteria.

Specifically, some owners are admitting persons who have a history of failure to pay rent in a timely manner, who cause damage to the premises, or who interfere with the enjoyment of the premises by other residents. The owner is free to reject applicants who display a history of any of the above mentioned traits. . . . Resident managers should not admit potential residents who will jeopardize the financial viability of the complex or who fail to respect either the premises or the rights of others.

Screening is the responsibility of the owner and housing manager. In developing screening policies and procedures, management must be sure that their policies and procedures comply with their obligations under Section 504 of the Rehabilitation Act of 1973 and Title VII of the Civil Rights Act of 1968 (Fair Housing Act).

In order to comply with the mandates of nondiscrimination, housing managers must be aware of the information that can and cannot be asked of housing applicants. According to a recent memo from the U.S. Department of Housing and Urban Development Region 1 Office (1991), housing managers may ask applicants about their

ability to comply with the terms of tenancy as set forth in the lease agreement. (For example, a landlord may ask about an applicant's ability to pay rent in a timely fashion or an applicant's ability to respect the rights and property of others.) This information should be uniformly solicited from all applicants. (U.S. Department of Housing and Urban Development, 1991, p. 1)

The memo goes on to specify areas that a housing manager may not ask of prospective tenants. According to the U.S. Department of Housing and Urban Development (1991, p. 1), a landlord **MAY NOT**:

- ask whether he or she has a disability or whether any member of the applicant's family or any friend or associate has a disability
- inquire about the nature or severity of any disability, nor ask any question that would require an applicant or tenant to waive the right to the confidentiality of a medical condition or medical history
- require the production of any medical records

Under certain circumstances, housing managers may ask questions about an applicant's disability. According to the U.S. Department of Housing and Urban Development (1991), questions regarding an individual's disability may be asked:

1. if disability is a prerequisite for eligibility for the housing;
2. if modifications are required to accommodate the individual's disability within the complex; or
3. if the normal screening procedures produce negative information about the individual's ability to meet the terms of the lease. (Under this last condition, procedures must be in place to assure the rights of *all applicants* to address the negative information derived from the screening process.)

Finally, according to the HUD guidelines: "A landlord should not attempt to assess whether an applicant is capable of independent living but only whether the applicant meets essential eligibility requirements" (U.S. Department of Housing and Urban Development, 1991, p. 2).

Standard screening criteria for subsidized housing include: (a) demonstrated ability to pay rent, (b) comments from previous landlords, (c) good credit references, and (d) housekeeping habits. Screening tools available to housing managers include: (a) use of credit checks, (b) landlord references, and (c) home visits. Information about prior landlords and credit history should be included in the application. Evidence of either a history of evictions or previous failures to pay rent provides documentation regarding an applicant's inability to meet the conditions of the lease. Applicants should provide three landlord references to enable the manager to judge whether problems have existed across several different living situations.

Home visits provide invaluable information. Careful observations during a home visit provide information concerning housekeeping habits, life-style, and indicators or signs of problem behavior (e.g., alcoholism, drugs, and so on). Knowledgeable observers can distinguish dwelling conditions due to normal wear and tear, landlord neglect, or failure to maintain the unit.

While inadequacies in any one area may not be sufficient to reject an elderly applicant, consistent evidence to support the

conclusion that the prospective tenant is unable to meet the conditions of the lease is grounds not to accept the tenant.

Housing administrators and managers must realize that their
actions in screening prospective tenants affect the character of the
tenant population and the overall housing environment. Increased
time and attention spent in screening reduce the number of problems over which the housing manager has no control.

Admission. The admission process provides an opportunity to
provide incoming tenants with information that clearly establishes the rights and responsibilities of both tenants and management in the housing. From the very beginning, management's
actions in conveying information to tenants should always seek to
safeguard the autonomy, freedom, and dignity of the individual
(Ambrogi, 1990). Therefore housing managers and their staff should
be aware of how their actions at the time of admission either foster
or impede the independence and autonomy of the tenant. The
following examples illustrate, on the one hand, positive interactions between incoming tenants and housing manager that foster
independence and, on the other hand, negative interactions that
function to subordinate and intimidate.

The housing manager at River Glen, an 80-unit senior housing complex, "interviews" all new tenants at the time of admission. The
interview, which lasts about 30 minutes, is intended to inform residents about the "**rules**" of the complex. The housing manager tells
residents about each rule and the consequences when a rule is violated.
She feels strongly that her time spent in orienting new tenants is very
beneficial because it reduces the number of problems that she encounters
with tenants. After a lengthy monologue enumerating the rules, the
manager concludes by asking the tenant if he or she has any questions.

At a second senior housing complex, Spring Green, the admission
process is very different. All new tenants meet with the housing
manager. The purpose of the meeting is to answer any questions the
new tenant might have, to inform the tenant of his or her rights and
responsibilities, and to provide information concerning the circumstances when a tenant may be transferred from the complex. The
discussion of tenants' rights is emphasized to foster the person's
sense of autonomy and independence. The orientation for the new
tenant also includes information about activities and structural pro-

visions for ensuring that tenants have maximum opportunities for involvement in decision making. Opportunities for leadership and participation in groups, such as the Tenant Council and others, are described. Tenants are encouraged to participate in all activities.

Each manager feels that she is "helping" elderly tenants to understand the rules and regulations of the housing complex and thereby easing the transition to the housing complex. The housing manager at River Glen, however, has missed an invaluable opportunity to involve the tenant from the very beginning and encourage autonomy and self-determination. In effect, her presentation to tenants stresses only the rules. New tenants hear a long litany of don'ts. As a result, from the very beginning the message conveyed is that in this place there is little respect nor is there any intention to facilitate autonomy.

To foster and encourage the autonomy and self-determination of each resident, the goals of the admission process should be to inform tenants of: (a) their rights and responsibilities, (b) management's rights and responsibilities, (c) safeguards for protecting tenants' rights, and (d) channels of communication for handling problems when they arise. At the time of admission, failure to clarify: the nature of the housing environment, the criteria for transferring a frail tenant, and the rights and responsibilities of tenants will inevitably lead to problems.

A helpful tool at the time of admission is the Personal Care Sponsor Statement. Each incoming tenant may be asked to designate a personal care sponsor. The personal care sponsor is asked to sign a statement that describes the expectations associated with this role. As a tool, however, it is only helpful if used properly. In many instances a Personal Care Sponsor Statement may be used either improperly or illegally. Therefore it is important to acknowledge how it cannot and should not be used. A Personal Care Sponsor Statement cannot be used as a requirement for admission. For elderly who are widowed and childless or isolated elderly, their inability to name a Personal Care Sponsor cannot be used to keep them from the housing. Admission cannot be delayed until a person is located who is willing to sign the Personal Care Sponsor Statement.

Second, when the topic of the Personal Care Sponsor is discussed with the new tenant, great care and sensitivity must be brought to the discussion. If handled improperly, requests for the tenant to designate a Personal Care Sponsor will foster dependence on the part of the elderly tenant. In explaining the purpose of the statement and the role of the sponsor, care should be taken to promote the autonomy and self-determination of the elderly tenant. Time should be spent in explaining:

- Why the statement is requested
- Under what conditions the sponsor would be contacted
- The rights of the tenant that protect the flow of information to the Personal Care Sponsor

Third, the tenant and the Personal Care Sponsor need to be informed that the statement is not legally binding and that the Personal Care Sponsor is not legally responsible for the elderly tenant.

Finally, if a Personal Care Sponsor Statement is incorporated into routine management practice, then the statement must be updated on a regular basis. Housing managers who fail to update their information on Personal Care Sponsors will inevitably find that the Personal Care Sponsor designated at the time of admission has moved, died, or is no longer available.

An example of a sponsor statement (Hamden Housing Authority, 1990) is as follows:

I _____ agree to be responsible for the care of _____. My responsibilities will include being the contact person in case of problems or emergencies regarding _____.

Furthermore, I understand that if _____ becomes incapable of independent living due to increased disability, either physically or mentally, I will assist (if I am requested) in relocating _____ to a facility better suited for his/her needs.

I understand that I am not responsible for any financial obligations. My responsibilities are assisting in the care of _____ when necessary.

Signature

Date

Other opportunities for providing information to tenants at the time of admission include: tenant orientation sessions and a tenant handbook. Tenant orientation sessions are a helpful way of conveying information about the housing. Informational sessions can be used to provide information concerning:

- Terms and conditions of the lease
- House rules
- Description of the recertification requirements
- Information about community services
- Opportunities for involvement in tenant organizations
- How to deal with problems when they emerge
- Getting to know staff

Resource materials can be developed for both tenants and personal care sponsors that provide information regarding services and resources available to older persons. A handbook for tenants should list rules and regulations, how to deal with various problems when they emerge, the right to appeal negative decisions, and channels of communication. A listing of regularly scheduled programs and activities included in the handbook provides encouragement for tenant participation.

Informational materials can also be developed for Personal Care Sponsors (Diehl, 1990). These materials should help them to:

- Promote the autonomy and self-determination of the older person
- Understand the importance of the support she/he provides
- Monitor changes in the tenant's behavior that may require some type of intervention
- Increase awareness and sensitivity to the needs of the older person
- Locate community resources should the need arise
- Understand normal changes that occur with aging

Retention and Relocation. The decision to relocate an elderly tenant is the most difficult decision that a housing manager must make. For the overwhelming majority of tenants, nursing home placement or a move to a more supportive residential environment is not perceived as a desirable option. Because frailty or disabilities threaten the older person's ability to live independently and meet the conditions of the lease, however, a decision must be made concerning a tenant's capacity to remain in independent housing.

As the previously discussed legal case involving the 90-year-old woman against senior housing management indicated, clear-cut policies concerning retention and relocation are essential for protecting the rights of both the tenant and the housing manager (Hellman, 1990). Retention and relocation policies must recognize simultaneously the needs and rights of elderly with disabilities and ensure the health and safety of all residents. Despite the importance of retention and relocation policies, several recent surveys of senior housing indicate that not all complexes have developed such policies. In fact, there is tremendous diversity across senior housing complexes concerning the presence and/or type of retention and relocation policies. Estimates of the percentage of housing complexes that have formal retention policies range from 92% (Suggs, Stephens, & Kivett, 1987) to less than half (Sheehan & Mahoney, 1984). A recent survey of large Public Housing Authorities (PHAs) reported that about 50% of the PHAs had formal retention policies (Holshouser, 1985; U.S. Senate, Special Committee on Aging, 1989). Of these, 10% require complete independence, approximately 30% retain residents who have some supportive service needs, while the remainder will retain residents if they or others can arrange for the necessary services. In a second study, roughly similar percentages of PHAs reported strict, moderate, and open criteria, respectively, for continued residence of elderly tenants (Sheehan, 1986a). According to this survey, 6% maintained strict criteria, 20% reported moderate (some supportive services), and 34% reported open criteria (any level of frailty or functional impairment as long as a tenant receives necessary supportive services).

While a component of any retention policy should be specification of procedures for assessing changes in functional level, most age-segregated housing environments do not collect relevant information on a regular basis. The previously discussed survey of large PHAs found that only about half of the housing authorities collected any type of information (e.g., residents' functional levels, medical histories, and use of services) on a regular basis (Holshouser, 1985; U.S. Senate Special Committee on Aging, 1989).

Ultimately, the decision to relocate an elderly tenant is necessitated when either the tenant lacks the necessary competence to meet the conditions of the lease or is unable to perform critical skills necessary for independent living *and* lacks adequate supportive services to assure his or her personal safety or the safety of others. Based upon recent legislation, functional disability is not a sufficient reason for relocation. The competence or frailty of the individual must be considered along with the availability of necessary supportive services.

"GOODNESS OF FIT" BETWEEN TENANT COMPETENCE AND ENVIRONMENT

Relocation decisions reflect a decision that the elderly tenant is no longer competent to remain in the particular housing environment. In other words, an appropriate "fit" no longer exists between tenant competence and the environment (Lawton, 1980; Lawton & Nahemow, 1973). To determine "fit," housing managers and social service providers need to assess both tenant competence (ability for survival, self-maintenance, and growth) and environmental demand (the nature of the demands that the environment places upon the individual). Competence extends across a number of areas of individual functioning: (a) health, (b) sensory-cognitive abilities, (c) capacity for self-care, (d) ability to perform instrumental activities, (e) mastery, and (f) social skills (Lawton, 1983).

Just as tenants differ in their overall competence levels, housing environments differ with respect to the demands they place upon tenants. Some environments are extremely demanding, while others put few demands on elderly tenants. At one end of the continuum are service-rich environments that provide for all their needs. In the extreme, they do not need to cook, clean, or even walk around. Everything is done for them. At the other end of the continuum are environments that provide no supportive services. When competence and environmental demands are matched—there is a "good fit." If the environment is too demanding for a tenant's competence or if the environment puts too few demands on a tenant's competence, there is a "poor fit" or mismatch. Typically housing managers and social service providers encounter situations in which the environment is too demanding for the competence level of the elderly tenant. If an excessively impaired tenant is allowed to remain in an environment that no longer meets his or her needs, the safety and well-being of the tenant and the other tenants are threatened. For the tenant, prolonged exposure to such a mismatched environment results in additional losses in functional ability and/or psychological well-being due to high levels of stress (Lawton, 1980; Lawton & Nahemow, 1973).

When a "poor fit" exists, managers may decide to: (a) relocate the tenant to a more supportive environment, (b) provide services to increase the supportive nature of the environment, (c) modify the physical environment to create a more supportive environment, or (d) do nothing. Housing managers may "do nothing" or fail to act for several reasons: (a) uncertainty concerning what to do, (b) perceived helplessness or past failures in efforts to relocate an elderly tenant, or (c) the belief that inaction is in the "best interests" of the tenant. Doing nothing, however, leads to further declines in a tenant's functional ability and well-being (Sheehan, 1986a).

For tenants in an environment that is too demanding, housing managers must either increase the supportive nature of the environment or relocate the tenant to a more suitable housing environment. While relocation should be the last resort, based upon the "goodness of fit" model, in many instances it can increase a tenant's functional competence and well-being if the demands of the new environment are more closely tied to the competence of the person. Thus, in certain circumstances when relocation becomes the only alternative, the elderly person may benefit from a move to an environment more closely suited to his or her needs.

When relocation becomes inevitable, housing managers must do everything possible to guard against the negative effects of relocation. Housing managers need to involve the tenant in the decision. Encouraging tenants to talk about what will happen and express their fears and concerns helps adjustment following the move. Tenants should be encouraged to exercise some control over the decision. Overly anxious or depressed elderly may be particularly stressed by the move. Efforts to help tenants deal with these feelings can ease the transition. Relationships with family and significant others can help ease the transition.

Housing managers should realize that the decision to relocate an elderly tenant does not represent failure on their part.

> Mr. Smith has been the Executive Director of a large housing authority for over 20 years. During this time he has instituted a variety of supportive service programs to maintain elderly tenants in their apartments. He takes great pride in the fact that he has never evicted an elderly tenant. During the past several months, however, an elderly tenant in one of Mr. Smith's senior housing complexes has suffered major problems that interfere with her ability to meet the conditions of the lease. Among the problems this tenant has experienced are significant deterioration in her ability to care for herself, incontinence, mental confusion, and inability to get around in her apartment.

Despite the Executive Director's efforts to bring in services, the tenant continues to evidence significant deterioration. Mr. Smith, however, refuses to seek relocation for this tenant. He takes great pride in the fact that in all his years working in elderly housing he has never moved to evict an elderly tenant. His reluctance to consider relocation, however, may lead to even more serious consequences.

Formal policies concerning retention and relocation help housing managers to make difficult decisions based upon a careful systematic determination that the tenant can no longer live in independent housing.

ASSESSMENT AS PART OF THE MANAGEMENT PROCESS

For social service providers, health care professionals, and housing professionals, the ability to assess accurately the circumstances of elderly tenants is essential. For many years social service and health care professionals have recognized the importance of assessment in developing care plans or intervention strategies for working with elderly tenants. As a result, social service and health care professionals have access to a wide variety of assessment tools to evaluate elderly clients. For housing managers, however, assessment, as part of their role, is a relatively recent issue to emerge. Consequently, there are few guidelines for how assessment in senior housing should be approached and only a limited number of assessment tools appropriate for use by housing managers.

Assessment Tools

Depending upon the particular type of assessment inventory, assessment can provide information concerning (a) the nature of the problem, (b) the cause of the problem, (c) what can be changed or modified to ameliorate the problem, or (d) whether the problem is serious enough to warrant intervention (Kane & Kane, 1981). In all cases, repeated assessments are essential for documenting changes that occur.

Selection of an appropriate assessment tool depends upon the person doing the assessment (e.g., educational background, degree and professional affiliation); the setting of the assessment (e.g., acute care hospital, adult day care setting, congregate housing or independent housing); and the reason for performing the assessment (Kane & Kane, 1981).

The remainder of this chapter focuses specifically on informal and formal assessment in senior housing.

Assessment in Senior Housing

Housing managers regularly assess or evaluate their elderly tenants. On a daily basis, housing managers determine who needs help, who may not be receiving adequate services, which families are no longer providing help, which tenants are in need of immediate intervention, when should a tenant be relocated, or when should a referral be made to a community service agency. These assessments reflect efforts to determine what is going on in the lives of elderly tenants, what problems are being experienced, and when a problem is serious enough to warrant intervention. Decisions or judgments about tenants, however, are most frequently based upon a housing manager's informal assessments. These informal assessments are based upon information derived from mental notes or recorded observations about a particular tenant.

What housing managers fail to realize is that there are a number of problems associated with this informal approach to assessment. First, if managers rely exclusively on memory or mental notes about tenants, they frequently make inaccurate judgments concerning what is really happening in an elderly tenant's life. Due to the limitations of human memory, housing managers are likely to forget significant aspects of behavior, engage in selective remembering, or be confused about when a particular problem behavior occurred. Written notes documenting changes in a tenant's behavior, functional level, or unmet needs are obviously far superior to mental notes about a particular tenant. Written observations provide a permanent record of problems or incidents that have occurred. These written observations, however, may be either unclear or confusing when later used to evaluate or judge an elderly tenant's behavior. The following excerpts taken from a housing manager's log indicate how entries about a tenant can be unclear or confusing:

12/9 Mrs. Jones appeared confused and disoriented at the monthly tenant meeting.
12/15 Mrs. Jones left a pot on the stove setting off the smoke detector.
12/29 Mrs. Jones fell on the sidewalk outside her apartment.

These entries concerning Mrs. Jones, however, lack objectivity and a standard against which the housing manager can judge Mrs. Jones's behavior. If Mrs. Jones appeared confused and disoriented, we need to know the extent and severity of her confusion. Was she disoriented: in knowing what to do? to place or time? or about who the other people were? The lack of a standard against which to judge particular behaviors can lead to unwarranted or inaccurate conclusions.

A second problem with this method is that the entries in a manager's log document behavior or behavioral changes for only tenants who get "noticed." While some tenants who are experiencing moderate to severe problems will be identified in this manner, a substantial number of vulnerable or "at risk" tenants are "invisible" and will not be recorded in a manager's log. For these tenants who fall through the cracks, opportunities for early intervention or remedial action are missed.

Finally, this method does not provide baseline data on all tenants. Because for older persons a significant change in functional status or behavior may be more indicative of potential problems than absolute level, systematic data concerning all tenants are needed. As a result, increased attention has focused on the role of formal assessment in senior housing.

Formal Assessment

Formalized assessment procedures in senior housing overcome many of the problems associated with informal assessment. Formal assessments provide a tool for guiding management decisions concerning tenants' ability to continue living in senior housing. If properly used, formal assessment can increase the options available to housing managers to deal with challenging situations, rather than limiting options about what to do when a tenant experiences problems associated with his or her disability.

In order to incorporate formal assessment into senior housing, a number of issues must be addressed. These issues include:

- The legal and ethical issues associated with assessment
- Criteria for determining suitability for continued residence
- Methods and tools for assessing functional status

Housing managers who desire to incorporate formal assessment procedures into their management role currently face a "Catch 22" situation. On the one hand, legal precedent has determined that housing managers can be judged liable if the decision is made to relocate an elderly tenant with disability without adequate documentation concerning a tenant's functional level. On the other hand, there are few legal protections for managers that support their rights to formally evaluate or assess tenants.

As a result, there is little agreement concerning the best way of incorporating formal assessment into the management role. In efforts to resolve the issue of assessment, housing managers must address the following questions:

1. Does the assessment violate a tenant's rights of privacy and self-determination?
2. What are the goals of the formal assessment?
3. Should all tenants be assessed or only those identified as having problems?
4. Should assessments be done on a regular basis or only when problems arise?
5. What aspects of functional competence are relevant or appropriate for the assessment?
6. Is assessment the responsibility of the housing manager or someone designated by the housing manager?

First and foremost, any assessment must protect the tenant's rights of privacy and self-determination. The ethical and legal implications of assessment in senior housing have yet to be fully explored.

Second, formal assessment must begin with a decision to evaluate certain aspects of behavior. For housing managers this decision will be guided by the guidelines or criteria for independent living that specify the minimum levels of functioning that all tenants must possess. In selecting an assessment tool, housing managers must select an instrument that evaluates *only* those competencies that directly relate to lease compliance.

In implementing formal assessment, procedural issues that housing managers must address include: (a) who will be assessed, (b) who will do the assessment, (c) when the assessment will be done, and (d) how the assessment will be done.

In establishing assessment procedures, housing managers must address the following issues:

1. Should all tenants be assessed to provide systematic information on all tenants or should only tenants experiencing problems be assessed?
2. Should assessments be done only when problems occur or periodically for all tenants?
3. Should the housing manager conduct the assessment or should responsibility be delegated to others?

Standardized Assessment Tools

Standardized assessment tools help managers to identify tenants with unmet needs, document systematic changes in tenants' levels of functioning, and identify tenants who are no longer appropriate residents in independent housing.

Currently, several assessment tools or approaches to assessment are available for use in senior housing. The three approaches discussed are Assessment of Independent Living Skills, developed by the Human Services Department of the Public Housing Agency of the City of Saint Paul; computerized case management assessment (Hellman, 1990); and screening.

Assessment of Independent Living Skills

The Assessment of Independent Living Skills, developed by the Human Services Department of the Public Housing Agency of the City of Saint Paul, is useful for assessing basic functional competencies of elderly tenants. The inventory evaluates 20 basic living skills. These skills are divided into 10 critical and 10 contributory factors.

The 10 critical factors are:

1. Meal preparation
2. Housekeeping
3. Mobility
4. Personal care (toilet)
5. Personal care (medications)
6. Orientation to time, place, and person
7. Decision making
8. Functional disorders
9. Alcohol/drug abuse
10. Safety awareness

The 10 contributory factors are:

1. Shopping
2. Financial
3. Transportation

4. Personal care (bathing)
5. Personal care (dressing)
6. Personal care (grooming)
7. Personal traits related to group living capabilities
8. Capability to maintain interpersonal relationships
9. Communication capabilities: hearing, sight, speech, and writing
10. Telephone communication capability

An adapted version of this instrument evaluates each of the 20 skill areas as either adequate or inadequate (Philbrick et al., 1991). (See Appendix A.) A skill area is judged adequate if the tenant is able to do it either without assistance or receives adequate help to perform. In evaluating each skill area, the basis of judgment/evidence should be noted. In some instances, the information is not available. This should be noted in the evaluation.

Guidelines for using the assessment indicate that critical factors relate to lease requirements and immediate health and safety conditions. If a resident's skill level in any of the critical factors is judged inadequate, serious consideration should be given to a supervised service-intensive living arrangement. If a person's skill level with supportive services is inadequate in more than one or two contributory factors, independent housing may not be advisable.

When making the final determination concerning a tenant's continued tenancy, additional factors need to be considered. These include the availability and appropriateness of supportive services and a tenant's willingness to accept services. The assessment should not be treated as an inflexible absolute from which there is no appeal. Extenuating circumstances, such as a tenant's willingness to accept supportive services or willingness of the family to provide services, should be weighted in making the decision concerning relocation. The Assessment of Independent Living Skills is a short, easy-to-administer assessment tool. The advantage of formalized assessment is that all tenants are judged against the same standards or criteria to determine their competence for independent living.

The assessment can be used regularly to determine tenants' continued appropriateness for independent senior housing. In subsidized housing the assessment can be included as part of the annual recertification process. This enables housing managers to make periodic assessments that document tenants' ability for independent living and any changes in functional ability that may signal the need for intervention. In private senior housing data may be collected as part of the annual conference held with the tenant and manager.

The advantages of regularized assessment are to: (a) provide routine systematic data on all tenants concerning their ability to function in independent housing, (b) document changes that have occurred from one year to the next, and (c) provide for objective documentation of functional ability.

The disadvantages are that it alone is insufficient to document changes that can occur suddenly in a tenant's level of functioning. In addition, a daily log should be maintained for documenting special problems that emerge. Information derived from the assessment does not indicate the underlying cause of a particular behavior. When a housing manager is concerned about a particular tenant, he or she may then choose to refer the tenant for a more detailed assessment.

Computerized Case Management Assessment

A second approach to assessment is a computerized case management assessment (Hellman, 1990). Use of this approach involves collection of baseline data at the time of admission with regular follow-up assessments to determine tenants needing additional attention. The criteria include: activities of daily living (e.g., bathing, grooming, toileting, mobility, meal preparation, etc.), incontinence, mental status, and social activity and social support (Hellman, 1990). Functional status on all components are rated using a 6-point scale (0 = least independent to 5 = most independent). The criteria are used to identify problem areas requiring intervention. (See Appendix B.) According to Hellman (1990), housing complexes should weight the criteria based upon their consequence for independent living. This approach provides an objective evaluation of elderly tenant's level of independent functioning. The overall functional status score derived from the assessment is similar to the APGAR score for newborns or global mental status evaluations (Hellman, 1990).

The proposed computerized model, however, does not provide specific directions for weighting individual dimensions of functional ability. According to Hellman (1990), "Each housing facility could customize the scoring as well as the criteria and assessment process" (p. 104). The assessment procedure provides a way of documenting changes that occur in tenants' behavior over a period of time and assuring prompt intervention.

Screening Approach

An alternative approach to assessment is screening. Screening uses a formalized reporting system whereby staff regularly observe tenant behavior. When a problem occurs, staff make a referral to the resident services coordinator or social service professional who does a comprehensive assessment. An example of this type of approach is an assessment procedure developed by the Westminster Company, a subsidiary of the Community Development Corporation of the Archdiocese of Saint Paul and Minneapolis, Minnesota (*Aging in place,* 1989). The screening procedures involve observation of five key behavioral indicators:

1. social
2. self-reliance
3. mental health
4. alcohol or drugs
5. physical health

Staff are trained to observe tenant behavior. If a staff member observes a change or decline in one of these areas, he or she documents the change through a formal report. As incidents/problems are observed, then a more comprehensive assessment is done to determine the nature of the problem.

Using this approach, only tenants displaying certain problems or declines are tracked within the system. Tracking of a tenant begins only after a staff member initiates a report. The advantages of this approach are that it is more time efficient and more responsive to changes in tenants' behavior because staff will report problems as they are observed. The major disadvantages of this approach are lack of baseline data on all tenants, failure to identify certain "invisible" tenants who are experiencing problems, rigorous training and monitoring of staff is needed to assure that all observations are recorded, and reliance on a resident services coordinator or other available professional to conduct the more comprehensive assessment. For housing managers, incorporating assessment into their routine management functions is increasingly important as more and more elderly tenants experience moderate to severe limitations in the ability to care for themselves. During the next several years, as the complexity of the challenges confronting housing managers increases, more attention will be directed to charting the course of assessment in senior housing.

CONCLUSION

During the past several decades it has become increasingly apparent that the management of senior housing presents special challenges. Effective housing management in senior housing directly contributes to the quality of life of elderly residents. Housing managers must be continually aware and vigilant in assuring that the needs of elderly tenants are met. Management of the physical plant, financial management, and facilitation of the social environment must be considered equally important functions that managers perform to assure the safety, security, and well-being of elderly tenants.

Residential policies concerning screening, admission, retention, and discharge provide tools for housing managers in planning for the inevitable changes that occur as elderly tenants age in place. Although frequently overlooked tools, thoughtfully developed policies are essential for assuring that the long-range goals of the housing complex are achieved. Further, policies provide helpful guidelines for housing managers in making difficult decisions that affect the overall operation of the housing complex.

Finally, the importance of assessment as part of the management role can no longer be ignored. Formalized assessment strategies provide housing managers with tools for decision making concerning the need for supportive services and the relocation of impaired tenants.

5

Physical Design and Quality
of Life in Senior Housing

$\mathbf{P}$HYSICAL design of the housing complex plays a major role in influencing the quality of life of all elderly tenants in senior housing. Consideration of design issues is particularly important for assuring that elderly persons with disabilities can live in the community with dignity and independence (Christenson, 1990; Pynoos, 1987). Housing managers, however, involved in the day-to-day demands of their jobs frequently overlook the importance of design as a key component of their management role. There are several reasons why housing managers pay little attention to design issues. First, many housing managers hold a narrow, static view of what is meant by design. They maintain that design refers exclusively to the objective physical features of the housing environment—size of the complex, layout, and availability of common spaces—features that are presumed to be constant or relatively unchanging. Following from this view, after a housing complex is designed and built, there is relatively little that a manager can do. Managers, therefore, either complain about a poorly designed complex or feel "blessed" to manage a well designed building. Second, housing managers may ignore design as part of their management role because they have received limited, if any, training concerning the impact of design and the environment on elderly tenants' well-being. Further, because many design issues such as privacy, security, controllability, and autonomy are elusive qualities, housing managers have difficulty in operationalizing these concepts.

This chapter, using a dynamic view of design and the physical environment, explores what housing managers and other professionals can do to create environments that foster and enhance elderly tenants' sense of security, competence, personal growth, and autonomy. Particular attention focuses on the role of design and the environment in the lives of elderly tenants with disabilities. Practical suggestions for modifying the environment are presented.

DESIGN AND THE ENVIRONMENT

Design is a dynamic concept extending beyond the physical dimensions of the built environment to include concepts such as safety, privacy, autonomy, order and predictability, and a sense of place and belonging (Pastalan, 1990). According to Pastalan (1990), aspects of design "do not flow automatically from well-designed spaces, but depend greatly on administration and staff" (p. 274). For example, privacy does not automatically occur because each tenant has his or her own apartment unit. Similarly, installation of a security system may not be sufficient to ensure that elderly tenants' needs for security are met. In other instances, the decision to provide extensive on-site services can conflict with efforts to promote autonomy and independence among elderly tenants. Failure to understand the more elusive qualities of design and the physical environment accounts for unsuccessful efforts to improve the quality of life of elderly tenants. For example, modifications or changes in the physical environment do not automatically guarantee the desired effect.

> Renovations to the community room at Hillview Senior Housing failed to increase the level of social activity and social interaction among elderly tenants. Despite newly painted walls, new furniture, improved lighting, and carpeting to improve the aesthetic quality of the common space, few tenants spend any time in the community room. The housing manager cannot understand why the improve-

ments in the physical environment have not increased tenants' shared social activity.

This housing manager failed to realize that the modification of the physical environment cannot be considered in isolation from the influence of the more elusive design factors on elderly tenants' behavior. To what extent do residential policies within the complex promote tenant self-determination and autonomy? To what extent do management practices encourage social interaction or social support among tenants? Therefore any suggestions concerning environmental modifications and changes must consider other factors that influence the behavior and well-being of elderly tenants.

Efforts to understand the complex interplay of design and the physical environment must begin by recognizing the interdependence between elderly tenants and their environment, the significant influence of management and staff on environmental quality and attributes, the relationship between environmental attributes and resident satisfaction, and the differential goals of environmental intervention.

Autonomy and Security: Dimensions of the Physical Environment

The most basic design issue that housing managers and designers must address in senior housing is the underlying tension between autonomy and security (Parmelee & Lawton, 1990; Pynoos, 1987). Housing managers who consider changing or modifying aspects of the environment should seek to achieve a reasonable balance between promoting safety and security and encouraging independence and autonomy (Parmelee & Lawton, 1990; Pynoos, 1987). Achieving a reasonable balance is critical because, say Parmelee and Lawton (1990), "overly secure environments produce boredom, apathy, and withdrawal; too much autonomy (i.e., in the absence of security) leads to stress and its documented effects" (p. 468).

As a general rule, designers, while acknowledging older persons' need for autonomy, place far greater emphasis on older persons' security needs (Parmelee & Lawton, 1990). Consequently, most suggestions or recommendations for improving the quality of the environment in senior housing focus primarily on the security/safety side of the issue. Much less attention has been directed at practical suggestions for increasing resident autonomy and self-determination. Recognizing this bias inherent in much design for older persons, housing managers, before implementing any suggested environmental modification, should consider the impact of this change on tenant autonomy. In other words, housing managers should consider what the "trade-offs" are between security and autonomy before a particular intervention or modification is put in place. Modifications of the physical environment should guard against possible negative effects on elderly tenants' psychological well-being and self-esteem. In efforts to increase the safety and security of senior housing, complexes should not be designed or modified to resemble mini-nursing homes. Rather, senior housing complexes should be designed and adapted to promote independent functioning among elderly tenants.

ADAPTATIONS OF THE PHYSICAL ENVIRONMENT

The following discussion of suggested adaptations of the physical environment focuses on interventions that promote the self-determination of elderly residents. Because most senior housing was not constructed to address the support needs of growing numbers of elderly tenants with disabilities, the proposed modifications seek to make senior housing environments more responsive and flexible to maximize elderly tenants' ability to care for themselves and to promote opportunities for personal growth and development. Estimates suggest that close to 50% of the elderly could benefit from modification of the physical environment (Struyk, 1987). These modifications can range from simple, relatively minor alterations to major structural changes.

Recommendations for environmental adaptations are divided into the desired outcomes of the intervention. These include: (a) removing physical barriers and/or impediments that interfere with tenants' ability to care for themselves, (b) implementing compensatory environmental changes to overcome sensory changes that occur with aging, (c) increasing the order and predictability of the environment to assist cognitively or emotionally impaired older adults in adapting to environmental demands, (d) rearranging physical spaces for increasing social interaction and social activity among tenants, (e) improving the aesthetic aspects of the environment to increase elderly tenants' morale or psychological well-being, and (f) eliminating hazardous environmental features to reduce the risk of accidents involving elderly tenants.

Removing Physical Barriers and/or Impediments

The overall intent of federal civil rights and fair housing legislation has been to ensure disabled persons full access to programs, services, and housing by removing barriers or impediments that have limited their full participation. More specifically, federal statutes—the Architectural Barriers Act of 1968 (ABA), Section 504 of the Rehabilitation Act of 1973, as amended, and the Fair Housing Amendments Act of 1988 (FHA)—all maintain disabled Americans' rights to achieve full access to programs and services. A key component of full access is the removal of architectural barriers and impediments. The three federal laws, however, establish different criteria for physical accessibility. Further, they apply differentially to various programs and situations. Under both Section 504 and the Fair Housing Amendments, physical accessibility is only one of several areas addressed to eliminate discrimination against persons with disabilities. Under the ABA, certain buildings financed by federal dollars must be accessible to disabled persons. Under this statute, the Uniform Federal Accessibility Standard (UFAS) sets the code or standard for how accessibility is to be achieved. Under Section 504, either the UFAS code or another standard that achieves equal or greater access can be used. The Fair Housing Amendments do not require full accessibility, but do require housing design to be adaptable for use by persons with disabilities. Standards for new construction include: accessible common spaces, adequate door widths to accommodate wheelchairs, accessible environmental controls (e.g., lights, thermostat, and so on), and usable kitchens and bathrooms to accommodate a person in a wheelchair.

The following example presents just one scenario of how these various standards apply under certain circumstances.

A Section 202 high-rise building will be occupied in May 1991. This building must comply with Section 504 because it receives federal funds. Under 504, 5% of the units must be accessible to persons with mobility impairments, and 2% of the units must be accessible to persons with visual or hearing impairments. The remaining units must meet FHA requirements as described in the Fair Housing Accessibility Guidelines or stricter standards. Under 540 and FHA, all public and common areas must be accessible.

Attention to issues of accessibility and adaptability is critical to the design of all elderly housing. In addition to the more stringent standards of accessibility for disabled persons, accessibility should be an overriding goal in all elderly housing. Design considerations should assure that living spaces promote elderly tenants' ability to move from one place to the other, to get in and out of spaces, and be unimpaired when attempting to carry out activities of daily living (Christenson, 1990). Design standards for elderly housing should create residential living spaces that are flexible and responsive to the need for older persons to live with dignity and independence. Accessibility standards should apply to all aspects of the built environment. For example, the design of closet and storage space and the selection of fixtures, such as light fixtures, door handles, and grab bars should reinforce and support older persons' ability to carry out activities of daily living (Christenson, 1990).

The goal of "adaptable housing" is to create environments that are flexible enough to meet the needs of elderly tenants with a wide range of functional levels and to meet the needs of elderly tenants as they age in place. Design features enable modifications of the physical environment to respond to elderly and disabled tenants' needs without major structural changes. Among the key design features of adaptable housing are: adjustable height counters and sinks, wider door widths, ground-level entrances, and work space to accommodate a person in a wheelchair (Christenson, 1990).

Implementing Compensatory Environmental Changes to Overcome Sensory Changes That Occur With Aging

With aging, significant changes in the vision and hearing of older persons alter the way in which they experience and perceive the environment (Christenson, 1990). Among the age-related visual changes that cause problems for elderly persons are structural changes affecting the lens of the eye, internal changes in the structure of the eye, and changes in the muscles that surround the eye. Due to changes in the transparency and thickness of the lens, older persons need increased light to be able to see (Christenson, 1990). As the lens becomes increasingly opaque, cataracts may begin to form so that by age 70 most older persons experience some problems with cataracts. The size of the pupil also decreases with age resulting in less light arriving at the retina. Similarly, changes in the muscles surrounding the eye and the elasticity of the lens are other normal changes that occur with aging.

As a result of these changes, older persons experience increased difficulty seeing, increased sensitivity to glare, blurred retinal images, and increased difficulty associated with adaptation when moving from bright light to indoor light (light-dark adaptation) (Christenson, 1990; Hiatt, 1987). As visual impairments increase, older persons may find it increasingly difficult to carry out many of their necessary daily activities. They may have difficulty in reading, writing out bills, telephoning, setting controls, finding lost objects, grooming, and preparing and eating meals. Problems also occur for visually impaired older persons in performing tasks such as shopping, laundry, housekeeping, and traveling. In addition, mobility activities such as driving become difficult, if not impossible, as a result of visual impairments (Hiatt, 1987).

Because for most older persons changes in vision occur over a long period of time, most develop strategies for coping with these changes (Hiatt, 1987). While many of these adaptive strategies are moderately effective in familiar surroundings, older persons with sensory deficits find it difficult to negotiate new, unfamiliar environments.

Within senior housing, a number of design modifications can be made to compensate for both normal aging-related visual changes and more serious impairments. Efforts to create a more responsive physical environment must begin with the realization, as Hiatt (1987) has noted, that, "The environment is not passive, it both aids and hinders visual and auditory competence" (p. 342).

The major types of interventions to improve older persons' ability to see their environment include: improving lighting quality, decreasing glare, improving legibility, and increasing contrasts between surfaces (Hiatt, 1987).

Glare Reduction

Despite older persons' need for increased light, too much light creates glare. Increased problems with glare are related to changes in the thickness of the lens and internal changes within the eye. Both direct and indirect glare present major problems for older persons. Sources of indirect glare that disturb older persons' visual ability include: light reflected off a highly polished floor, bright sunlight reflecting through large picture windows, plastic covering on furniture, or light reflecting off any shiny or glossy surface.

Practical suggestions for reducing problems associated with glare include (Christenson, 1990; Hiatt, 1987):

Avoid using glossy paint or shiny plastic tabletops

Use shades, blinds, or other window treatments to reduce bright sunlight reflecting through windows

Choose floor covering without shiny finishes

Cover windows with glare-reducing film

Install indirect lighting

Use nonglare glass and surfaces covering signs

Plant trees for shade to reduce glare

Install fluorescent light fixtures combined with incandescent lights to increase lighting

Use focused task lighting

Remove translucent wall light fixtures

Use posters/signs printed on matte surfaces

Increased Lighting

Due to normal aging-related visual changes, older persons need two to three times more light than younger persons to accomplish tasks successfully (Hiatt, 1987). Because of older persons' increased sensitivity to glare, however, the solution is not simply to replace lights with higher wattage bulbs (Blank, 1991). Rather, the solution is to locate lighting in key areas that maximizes older persons' visual capacities.

First, lights should be focused on work areas to provide necessary increased illumination to accomplish the task. Examples of locations for improved lighting sources include: dining tables, arts and crafts tables or surfaces, handrails in hallways and the illumination of signs (Hiatt, 1987). In some instances certain tasks require increased levels of illumination.

Well-maintained and good-quality fluorescent lighting in conjunction with incandescent lighting provides an excellent lighting source where high levels of illumination are needed, such as bathrooms (Christenson, 1990). When using fluorescent lighting, however, care should be taken to assure that lighting fixtures spread the light evenly (Christenson, 1990). Proper maintenance of fluorescent lights is also essential to eliminate problems caused by flickering (Hiatt, 1987). According to Hiatt (1987), "All fluorescent and incandescent light should be indirect. This means that bulbs should not be visible to the user" (p. 363). Lamp shades, valances, and other methods of diffusing light are essential for shading light from the direct line of vision. Lighting in corridors, hallways, and stairs should provide sufficient illumination to avoid falls and other accidents. The placement of light fixtures in these areas should provide maximum, continuous illumination. Care should be taken to avoid shadows or other breaks in the lighting that can lead to accidents or falls (Hiatt, 1987). To minimize glare light fixtures in hallways or corridors should not be placed at eye level (Hiatt, 1987).

Improved Contrasts

In addition, the use of contrasts in designing or modifying senior housing environments is crucial for older persons' ability to see objects well and discriminate objects (Christenson, 1990). Attention to eliminating glare and improving lighting is not sufficient for improving elderly tenants' ability to discriminate objects (DiStefano & Ashton, 1986). The effective use of color, depth, intensity, outline, size, and textures helps older tenants distinguish objects or surfaces from their backgrounds and thereby improves the functional visual abilities of elderly tenants. In many instances, contrast may be more important than illumination in assuring older persons' optimal visual functioning.

Changes in the lens of the eye alter the quality of light reaching the pupil and older persons' perception of certain colors. As a result, older persons have difficulty differentiating among different colors or shades. For example, many older persons may be unable to distinguish among pastel colors, such as yellows, beiges, pinks and so on. Therefore rooms, hallways, or activity spaces that are painted in different pastel colors to provide sensory cues to older persons are ineffective for most older persons (Hiatt, 1987).

Given aging-related losses in the ability to distinguish certain colors, contrasting colors should be used to demarcate certain areas or surfaces. For example, color contrast should be used to designate the handrail and the wall, wall and floor, wall and door floor and stairs. According to Christenson (1990), "When designing living situations for the elderly, the goal in color design is not only to make an area more aesthetically pleasing, but also to help contrast different areas or to be able to distinguish objects from their backgrounds" (p. 12). Alterations in textures may also be used to distinguish areas within the environment.

The use of contrasting color or tape to outline areas helps older persons to discriminate objects from their background and improves their depth perception. Simple modifications to improve contrasts in senior housing include placing contrasting tape around light sockets, painting door frames with contrasting colors to distinguish them from walls, use of contrasting color tape at the edge of steps, and selection of a dark rug to contrast with light furniture (DiStefano & Ashton, 1986).

Use of patterns in floor coverings should also be avoided (Christenson, 1990; Hiatt, 1987). Patterned floor coverings may be particularly distracting for older persons who experience problems with depth perception. Figures or patterns on the floor may appear as objects to walk around or step over. A sudden step to avoid an "object" on the floor may increase the likelihood of serious falls.

Use of signs or graphics to orient or inform elderly tenant should also reflect consideration of the normal visual changes that occur with aging. Important guidelines for using signs or graphics in elderly housing include (Hiatt, 1987): lettering on signs should have a contrasting background, use simple lettering to increase legibility, size of lettering should be large enough to enhance readability and proportional to the distance from which it is read and signs should never be printed on a glossy surface or encased behind a glass cover.

Thoughtful attention should be directed at the use of graphics in senior housing. According to Hiatt (1987), if graphics are used to designate certain areas or to serve as orienting devices, they should be representational rather than abstract symbols. Christenson (1990), however, cautions that inappropriate use of graphics may create an institutional, rather than homelike feeling, in the residential complex.

For visually impaired older persons, low vision aids are available to help compensate for vision losses. Aids include: large type reading materials, large easy to read telephone dials, and magnifying glasses.

Aging-Related Decrements in Hearing

Most older persons suffer some loss or deterioration in their hearing ability. The most common type of hearing loss that occurs during old age is presbycusis. *Presbycusis* refers to damage that affects the nerve endings and auditory hair cells in the inner ear. One of the major consequences of presbycusis is difficulty in hearing high frequency sounds (e.g., whistles, fire alarms, etc.). Further, older persons who suffer some type of hearing loss are increasingly susceptible to the disruptive effects of background noise. For many older persons, background noise interferes with the ability to hear and actively participate in normal conversations. Excessive background noise has also been linked to increased accidents and falls.

A number of modifications of the physical environment are suggested to create environments that maximize older persons' ability to hear and reduce the risks of accidents due to disruptive background noises. These include use of: acoustical ceiling tile, carpeting, draperies, and wall hangings to absorb unwanted background noise (Christenson, 1990). Such modifications of the physical environment also serve to create a more homelike, personal environment.

In addition, special insulating sheetrock can be used to muffle sounds coming from particularly noisy areas (Christenson, 1990). It is important to point out, however, that the goal of acoustical modifications should not be the elimination of all noise. Noise associated with certain areas (e.g., dining rooms, community rooms) can provide an important orienting cue for elderly tenants (Christenson, 1990).

Finally, as a safety feature, all smoke detectors and fire alarms should be combined with visual cues to ensure the safety of hearing-impaired elderly tenants (Christenson, 1990).

Increasing Order and Predictability

Environmental interventions to increase order and predictability in the environment assist cognitively impaired tenants in negotiating and finding their way in their housing complex. Particular attention should be directed to analyzing the "legibility" of the environment to assist tenants in understanding the various subcomponents of the environment. Multistory housing complexes with long corridors all painted the same color do little to either orient elderly tenants or reduce ambiguity. Environmental strategies to help elderly tenants comprehend aspects of the environment involve the provision of cues and landmarks that designate specific areas (Christenson, 1990). Tenants should be encouraged to personalize their doors. This strategy not only assists elderly tenants in differentiating their door from those of other tenants, but also enables tenants to select meaningful decorations that provide a sense of personal identity and continuity with the past.

Color coding or cueing alone does not provide sufficient information to enhance the readability of the environment. Special landmarks, such as grandfather clocks, large potted plants, large pictures, and so on, increase the safety of the environment and improve elderly tenants' ability to understand and negotiate within the complex (Christenson, 1990).

The personalization of doors and the selection of meaningful objects to serve as landmarks not only increase the legibility of the housing environment, but also enhance elderly tenants' sense of belonging. Further, using personally meaningful environment cues or landmarks reduces the institutional appearance of senior housing complexes.

Rearranging Physical Spaces for Increasing Social Interaction and Social Activity Among Tenants

Physical and design features of senior housing influence opportunities for social interaction and support, however, it is important to point out that physical design alone is not sufficient to reduce problems of social isolation and inactivity. Management policies and the actions of staff are *more important* than the physical environment (Cranz, 1987; Pynoos, 1987). In the words of Cranz (1987), "The solution to problems of social isolation is best met through innovations in social programming and not through physical design alone" (p. 98).

Among the features of the physical environment that may influence opportunities for social interaction are: size, layout, common spaces, and attractiveness. Although the relationship between complex size and level of social activity among elderly tenants is equivocal, there is some evidence to suggest that larger complexes are associated with more social isolation (Christensen & Cranz, 1987) and interpersonal conflict (Timko & Moos, 1990). Tenants residing in larger complexes are less likely to engage in mutually supportive relationships with other tenants, know fewer tenants by sight, and are less likely to form close personal friendships with other tenants (Christensen & Cranz, 1987).

Within larger housing complexes, several strategies to break down barriers that prevent social interaction and increase interpersonal conflict can be implemented. First, creation of smaller, meaningful residential units, such as "neighborhoods" creates a sense of social awareness of one's neighbors and fosters a sense of community. Regular neighborhood social activities and monthly meetings provide opportunities for tenants to get to know one another and to express specific concerns about their floor. Second, outreach efforts by a social worker can break down barriers to social interaction by increasing tenants' perceptions of the common bonds they share (Christensen & Cranz, 1987). Third, strategically located common areas on each floor provide a locus for informal socialization among neighbors outside of individual apartments. Finally, improved channels of communication between tenants and staff reduce interpersonal conflict and alienation in larger complexes (Timko & Moos, 1990).

Common spaces or activity spaces provide opportunities of social interaction among tenants, however, the availability of common space does not guarantee that social activities and social interaction will occur (Regnier, 1987). Suggestions for improved utilization of common spaces come from environmental design and postoccupancy studies (Regnier, 1987). Common spaces adjacent to the lobby and located strategically near the hub of activity provide tenants opportunities for developing familiarity with the space before committing themselves to participation. Common social spaces located near a heavily traveled route will be more frequently used than out of the way, secluded areas (Regnier, 1987). Whether used for a meal program, group activities, or community events, centrally located common spaces are critical for the social life of the housing complex. Common spaces should provide opportunities for tenants to preview the area (Regnier, 1987). Spaces behind closed doors do little to invite potential new participants.

Lobbies in senior housing are one of the most controversial topics to be discussed. Some managers refuse to allow tenants to sit in the lobby, while others feel that lobbies are an important part of the social life of the complex. Research has documented both the positive and negative impact of lobbies on elderly tenants' psychological well-being and levels of social interaction. On the positive side, lobbies offer elderly tenants opportunities for informal socializing, observation, and keeping up to date on current events. Further, larger lobbies have been shown to be related to higher levels of social interaction among elderly tenants (Christensen & Cranz, 1987).

Lobbies, however, can be a source of tension and difficulty for some elderly tenants. For nosy people, lobbies provide an excellent vantage point for sitting and watching the comings and goings in the complex. Carp's (1987) research describing elderly public housing tenants' experiences noted many tenants' complaints about "lobby sitters" who gossip about everyone coming through the lobby. Our own experience in conducting interviews with elderly tenants in federally assisted housing noted how "lobby sitters" who gossip about other tenants disrupt some tenants' ability or comfort in pursuing their everyday activities. One elderly tenant who complained about the gossip and busybodies who keep track of everybody's business told an interviewer that she collects her mail from the lobby at 2:00 a.m. to avoid being seen by these gossipy tenants. In other instances, says Cranz (1987), policies have been established to prohibit persons from sitting in the lobby "based upon aesthetic anxiety" (p. 84).

Given the controversy surrounding lobbies in senior housing, much thought and attention must be directed to how policies and the physical design of the lobby and means of accessing the housing environment operate to facilitate social interaction. First, management policies must respect the dignity and independence of all elderly tenants. Gossip, bickering, and other types of social interaction should not be ignored; rather, sources of negative interactions must be addressed to ensure tenants' rights to age in place with dignity. Management and staff serve as role models for promoting interactions that treat everyone with dignity and respect.

Second, lobbies should be designed to maximize the benefits and minimize the costs associated with lobbies. One of the benefits of lobbies is the provision of increased opportunities for social interaction. To achieve this desired effect, lobbies should be large enough to handle the heavy flow of traffic. When mailboxes are located in the main lobby of the complex, increased opportunities for social interaction among elderly tenants are provided (Cranz, 1987). Tenants gradually come to know other tenants by sight from having seen them repeatedly in the lobby area. For tenants who are reluctant initially to get involved with other tenants, a central lobby provides a vantage point or surveillance zone to view the social life of the housing complex (Regnier, 1987). Despite the purported advantages of central mailboxes, however, some elderly tenants complain that mailboxes are "too public" (Carp, 1987). Housing managers should decide based upon the social climate in their housing (e.g., level of gossip, social conflicts, etc.) the best location for mailboxes and mail drops in their buildings.

Finally, because all design should promote tenant autonomy and self-determination, senior housing should provide an alternative entrance to tenants who desire to avoid the central lobby.

Simple modifications can lead to real changes in the ways common spaces are utilized. For instance, redecorating common areas (e.g., comfortable chairs, newly painted bright walls, etc.) can increase the ambience and attractiveness of these areas to promote social interaction. Rearranging furniture in common areas increases opportunities for informal social interaction. Comfortable chairs should be arranged in small groupings to facilitate opportunities for conversation. Creating a less institutional, more home-like environment increases the desire for pleasant interactions with other tenants.

Reallocation of space to common areas, adding additional space, or modifying existing space (e.g., glass window walls to preview activities) all serve to invite social participation and increase tenants' motivation to participate in social activities. Decisions regarding the use of space by various community groups or programs need to be made carefully. Shared areas between residents and the community create potential conflicts over space.

As a general rule, inconvenient, inaccessible, or unattractive common spaces do little to facilitate social interaction. Complexes that offer tenants more comfort features (e.g., attractiveness, space, and convenience) increase mutual support, cohesion, and tenant self-determination and independence (Timko & Moos, 1987). Logically, feeling good about one's home and a sense of pride promote both a sense of belonging and independence among elderly tenants.

Consideration of common spaces for purposes of increasing opportunities for social interactions should take into account outdoor areas as well as interior spaces (Regnier, 1987). Well-designed outdoor spaces provide invaluable opportunities for facilitating social interaction. Attractive benches and other seating arrangements, strategically located, encourage elderly tenants to get out of their apartment to enjoy the fresh air with their neighbors.

Efforts to increase social interaction and support among elderly tenants, however, will be futile unless corresponding attention is directed to management policies and the actions of staff. Housing managers should realize that social structures and management policies are more important than structural change in achieving increased levels of social activity and social interaction. Social structures, such as tenant councils and innovative social programming, are major design factors that influence social interaction and social activity among elderly tenants.

Improving the Aesthetic Aspects of the Environment

Living in an attractive, well-maintained senior housing complex is related to elderly tenants' satisfaction with their housing (Butterfield & Weidemann, 1987). Housing managers should strive to create a pleasant, homelike environment for elderly tenants. The choice of colors, furniture, and decorations is important not only to compensate for aging-related decrements, but also to achieve a pleasant living environment. The very appearance of common spaces can do a great deal either to attract or to repel elderly tenants from participating in planned activities.

Attractiveness of the physical environment is a major factor that contributes to resident satisfaction. Tenants' overall satisfaction with the attractiveness of their complex is related to such factors as: a homelike setting, a pleasant community building, appropriate interiors, ease of finding their way around the complex, special recreational facilities, and a noninstitutional appearance on the exterior. Housing managers should strive particularly to facilitate a homelike atmosphere in senior housing. In addition to the decor, a homelike atmosphere is provided when tenants' feel a sense of ownership of the facility (Butterfield & Weidemann, 1987). The means of achieving a sense of ownership include assigned parking spaces and circulation routes that do not allow outsiders to intrude into tenants' space.

Encouraging tenants to personalize the environment also facilitates a sense of ownership. Tenants should be allowed to maintain control over their home spaces. Too much rigidity and an homogenized environment stifle individuality and present a sterile picture or image of the people who live in the housing, while variation from one unit to the next both underscores the individuality of elderly tenants and increases environmental cues for way finding and orientation. Tenants should be encouraged to have input concerning the exterior image of the housing environment. Input regarding landscaping and other aspects of the site should reflect tenants' desires concerning the public image of their housing complex. The selection of trees, shrubs, and other outside amenities increases the attractiveness of the housing and conveys a message about the tenants who live there (Butterfield & Weidemann, 1987).

Attractiveness is also related to the use of quality materials. The use of materials symbolizes the "value" that society places on the inhabitants. If building materials are not of high quality, the message conveyed underscores the societal stereotype that older persons are not valued members of society. Attractiveness is also related to the level of maintenance in senior housing (Butterfield & Weidemann, 1987).

The provision of physical amenities such as social recreational spaces, personal spaces, and so on, also increases the attractiveness of the housing complex. Elderly tenants who live in senior housing complexes that provide a variety of physical amenities are significantly more satisfied than tenants who live in accommodating housing.

Overall, housing managers should realize that careful, thoughtful attention to the design, construction, maintenance, and management policy aspects of the environment is critical for improving tenants' satisfaction with and sense of belonging associated with their housing. For elderly tenants, the development of a sense of belonging is not likely to develop when the complex is poorly maintained. Broken windows, ripped screens, faded exteriors, or littered grounds alienate older persons from feeling a sense of connectedness with the housing environment.

Elimination of Hazardous Environmental Features

Finally, environmental planning, design, and monitoring of the physical plant should provide safe and secure environments that reduce or eliminate the risk of accidents or falls. Many of the suggestions discussed above to modify aspects of the physical environment also reduce or eliminate hazardous elements of the environment. For example, improved lighting and reduced background noise can significantly reduce the risk of falling and other accidents.

Housing managers should be aware of other potentially hazardous areas or conditions in senior housing that can lead to falls or accidents. Environmental risks or hazards that should be addressed immediately include: unsecured rugs or scatter rugs, lack of railings on stairs, uneven surfaces on floors, stairs or walkways, and low beds and toilets (Pynoos, 1987).

Everyone knows how dangerous kitchens can be. A number of design modifications can eliminate or reduce significantly the number of accidents that happen in the kitchen. For example, stoves should be equipped with automatic shut-off devices and large dials for ease of vision and manipulation (Regnier, 1987). Tenants prefer controls located on the front of the stove (Carp, 1987; Cranz, 1987). Some of the problems related to the placement of controls at the back of the stove are described in the following quotes from elderly tenants: "I'll have to be awful careful leaning over the hot burner to turn it off. I can't hardly see back there where you have to turn things" (Carp, 1987, p. 59). Controls should not only be easy to reach but also identifiable by sight and touch (Cranz, 1987).

Adequate task lighting in both the kitchen and bathroom are also particularly important safety interventions (Butterfield & Weidemann, 1987). The provision of slip-resistant surfaces in both the kitchen and bathroom can also reduce the likelihood of serious falls (Christensen & Cranz, 1987).

As previously noted under part of the routine management function, a wide range of management activities are critical to ensuring safety. As part of their management function, housing managers should:

- Monitor surface areas, such as walkways, paths, stairs for uneven surfaces that can lead to falls
- Monitor lighting and replace light bulbs to assure adequate lighting
- Make sure surface areas and circulation routes are free of obstacles that interfere with elderly tenants' ability to move freely around the complex
- Check that furniture is firm and steady (because wobbly or unsteady furniture can lead to falls)
- Make sure outside night lighting is adequate to ensure both the safety and security of elderly tenants
- Provide adequate storage space that is easily accessible to elderly or disabled tenants
- Make sure that aspects of the physical environment that older persons must manipulate or move are easily movable (e.g., doors should not be too heavy or difficult to open)

CONCLUSION

Environmental research strongly supports the benefits of environment manipulation for the safety, autonomy, psychological well-being, and social connectedness of elderly tenants. If housing managers assume a proactive stance toward the environment, numerous opportunities exist for enhancing the quality of life of elderly tenants.

Housing managers need to identify possible ways in which the environment can make it possible for elderly tenants to function at their maximum capabilities. High expectations and challenging environments provide opportunities for growth and personal development for older tenants. As Moos, Lemke, and David (1987) state, creating environments "that treat older persons as responsible adults" (p. 197) enhances residents autonomy and self-determination. Environments that are too protective can rob an elderly tenant of feelings of competence and vitality.

While admittedly not easy to create senior housing complexes that balance autonomy and security, the numerous benefits for elderly tenants' psychological, social, and physical well-being make it worth the difficulty.

6

Building a Positive Social Environment
in Senior Housing

FOR housing managers responsible for the operation of any type of communal living situation, the reality of group living is that it is both a blessing and a bane. On the one hand, it provides the opportunity to create a sense of community that links older persons together and fosters a sense of identity and connectedness. On the other hand, communal living involves the potential for deep-seated and long-lasting interpersonal conflicts and disagreements among tenants (Ryther, 1987). Typical problems that housing managers confront involve aspects of the social environment. Frequent bickering, gossip, apathy, or low levels of social activity are all reflections of the social environment. Similarly, lack of family support, family overprotectiveness, and family anger and resentment reflect problems of the social environment that extend beyond the immediate housing environment.

This chapter focuses on ways of building a social environment that promotes social interaction and positive self-esteem among elderly tenants. It is designed to equip housing managers and social service and health care professionals with basic knowledge concerning social interaction and social support and strategies for modifying the environment to enhance the well-being of elderly tenants.

DIMENSIONS OF THE SOCIAL ENVIRONMENT

The social environment includes obvious features such as the people with whom we interact, those with whom we share our thoughts and secrets, those we love, and those who help us with our everyday tasks: our spouse, our children, our friends, and our neighbors. Our interactions with these people can make us feel loved, important, or supported. In other instances our interactions can make us feel dependent, unloved, uncared for, and unhappy.

Successful strategies for fostering a positive social environment rest upon an understanding of the multidimensional nature of the environment and the complex patterns of interactions that make up the social environment.

SOCIAL ENVIRONMENT IN SENIOR HOUSING

The social environment exists at three levels: the housing complex, the local community, and the society at large. Within the housing complex, dimensions of the social environment include: the social climate; levels of social activity, interaction, and participation; social status norms and hierarchy involving elderly tenants, staff, and others; formal and informal expectations concerning appropriate behavior, such as visiting, helping, gossiping, and so on; and the presence and availability of informal and formal support.

At the local-community level, the social environment is influenced by community attitudes toward old age and senior housing; the flow of people, resources, and services from the community to the complex; the availability of community-based formal support services; and family support and values, attitudes, and behaviors.

Finally, at the societal level, it consists of events, values, and beliefs that have an impact on tenants and staff; public policies and legislation that affect housing and older persons; and overall social attitudes and values.

Events that occur in the community and the larger society have an impact on the social life in the housing complex. Similarly, events that occur within the complex have consequences that extend beyond the immediate environment. Change in the social environment may, therefore, originate at any one of the three levels.

Interventions aimed at improving the social environment may be aimed at altering social processes or dynamics at the level of the housing complex, the community, or, because the elements of the system are interrelated, at the broader society.

SOCIAL WORLD OF ELDERLY TENANTS

Efforts to create a warm positive environment in senior housing must begin by recognizing tenants' perceptions of the social environment, their desires for social activity, and the quality of tenant interactions and social support. In their efforts to plan and organize activities for tenants, housing managers frequently make inaccurate assumptions about older persons' desires for social activity that reflect the housing managers' own needs and desires. As Carstensen (1987) states, however, "The assumption that 80-year-olds desire the same social worlds as 40-year-olds is probably as erroneous as the assumption that 10-year-olds have the same social goals as 30-year-olds" (p. 224).

Tenants' Perceptions of the Social Environment

The first step toward building a positive social environment is to understand how elderly tenants perceive the social environment (Timko & Moos, 1990).

Housing managers should ask themselves:

- Do tenants perceive the environment offering opportunities for independence and self-determination?
- Do housing rules and regulations encourage social participation?
- How stimulating or boring do tenants view the environment?
- Is the housing staff perceived of as supportive and helpful?
- Are other tenants viewed as helpful and friendly?

Without shared consensus between the housing staff and tenants, efforts to build a more supportive environment will be unsuccessful.

When significant differences between the perceptions of the housing manager and tenants exist, problems related to the social environment will inevitably occur. While there is some evidence to suggest that there is moderate agreement between housing managers' and tenants' perceptions of the social climate (cohesion, conflict, independence, and resident influence) (Timko & Moos, 1990), other research suggests that housing managers overestimate the levels of sociability and social support among elderly tenants (Sheehan, 1986b). If housing managers overestimate the extent of mutual support among tenants, they are less likely to perceive unmet social needs among tenants. If housing managers understand how elderly tenants perceive the social environment, then chances of improving the quality of life of elderly tenants are increased.

Changes in Social Activity and Social Participation

Tremendous diversity characterizes the social lives of older persons. While most older persons experience declines in social activity due to loss of social roles, limitations in physical functioning, and loss of social relationships, a small group of elderly actually increase their activity as they age (Carstensen, 1987).

Older persons interpret changes in their social activity very differently. For some, declines in social activity represent increased freedom from obligatory roles and responsibilities. For others, decreased levels of social activity represent a coping strategy to conserve energy in the face of declining health and functional ability. In either case, the decline is not necessarily detrimental to psychological well-being.

The following brief case study illustrates how decline in social activity is perceived positively, as a well-deserved reward.

Mrs. R, age 72, is a widow and the mother of 10 children. She moved to a senior housing facility 3 years ago. Her health is good and she does not experience any impairments in her ability to care for herself. Since her move, she has dramatically reduced her level of social activity. She is completely satisfied with her low levels of social activity. In her own words, "No kids, no worries, no work."

For other elderly tenants, loss of social activity is undesirable and associated with feelings of loneliness and social desolation. Among these lonely elderly tenants, some strongly desire to replace lost social roles and activities; but they lack the necessary skills, resources, and/or opportunities to engage in new activities or establish new relationships. In other instances lonely elderly tenants feel that available activities are not "meaningful" to replace lost activities.

Several case studies illustrate poignantly the experiences of lonely elderly tenants. Reasons for their loneliness include loss of friends through death or relocation, changes in the perceived social environment ("tenants are not as friendly and outgoing as they used to be"), inability to participate actively in social activities, and lack of meaningful relationships (Sheehan & Mahoney, 1984).

Mrs. N

Mrs. N, age 74, is a widow. She was one of the original in-movers to a public senior housing complex 12 years ago. According to Mrs. N, over the years, she has decreased her level of social activity and become less involved with her neighbors. Presently she has little contact with any of her neighbors. According to Mrs. N, in the past the tenants "seemed more friendly and outgoing when I first moved in. The tenants are not as friendly as they used to be."

Mrs. C

Mrs. C, an 81-year-old widow, is badly crippled. Mrs. C's attitude toward aging is reflected in her remark that when she reached 80 she was "old." And now at 81, Mrs. C has lived in public senior housing for the past 12 years. Presently her social activities with her neighbors are extremely limited. Describing her social relations, Mrs. C noted, "I talk to everybody and people are nice enough . . . but to be a real friend I can't be . . . I can't especially now go anywhere with . . . but before when I could go, I went on a few trips before, but now I can't." A widow for the past 26 years, Mrs. C reports that as she gets older she misses her husband more and more. When she was hospitalized several months ago, she believed that she would "meet her husband." Although Mrs. C sees her daughter regularly, has regular contact with two of her sisters, and limited contact with several tenants, she is very lonely sometimes.

Mrs. D

Mrs. D, a widow for the past 19 years, indicated that she began to feel lonely after her mother died in 1975. During her life, Mrs. D spent 15 years caring for her husband's grandfather, 10 years caring for her husband following his stroke, and most recently 3 years caring for her mother. Mrs. D reported that she used to go to the senior center but "got so tired of playing bingo" that she does not go anymore.

Mrs. A

Mrs. A, a 79-year-old widow, is very lonely and suffering from depression for which she is under a psychiatrist's care. She has lived in senior housing for the past 9 years. According to Mrs. A, she had friends when she first moved to the senior complex, however, several have gone to a convalescent home, and one died. Her social contact consists of limited contact with her next door neighbor and a "telephone friend" who calls her occasionally.

Mr. B.

Mr. B, an 84-year-old widower, prides himself on his independence. While he noted that he has made a "lot of friends . . . and it's a nice atmosphere. . . . They keep their distance and so do I." While he prides himself on his ability to cook, clean and do laundry, he admitted "I'd like to have some company though . . . but . . . I can get along without that too."

A small group of elderly tenants actually increase their levels of activity as they age (Carp, 1987). For these elderly, their new-found freedom enables them to engage in a wide variety of activities such as senior center activities, social clubs, and volunteer work. Other elderly tenants who have led socially isolated lives throughout their adult lives continue their previous life-style patterns and preferences.

Is Social Activity a Prescription for Positive Mental Health?

Most housing managers assume either explicitly or implicitly that high levels of social activity reduce feelings of loneliness. For many, the prescription for positive mental health is "Be Active." While there is some evidence that elderly tenants who participate in formal activities report higher levels of psychological well-being, studies of elderly persons in the general population do not consistently support this conclusion (Carstensen, 1987). "Activity" includes involvement with family, friends, and neighbors; participation in formal organizations such as senior centers; educational pursuits; fraternal/ethnic organizations, and so on; and leisure activities such as playing cards and/or bingo. Not all activities reduce feelings of loneliness.

Older persons' assessment of the adequacy of their social relations and activities is more important to well-being than either the frequency or number of their activities. Stated in other words, it is the perceived quality not the frequency of social involvement that contributes to well-being. Of all activities, relationships with companions and confidants are most directly related to improved psychological well-being (Chappell & Badger, 1990).

In contrast to the assumption that activity, in and of itself, is a goal, housing managers should view planned activities as a means of achieving certain goals. Take time to reflect about your attitudes concerning activities, the activities offered at your housing complex, and possible future programs.

1. What are your personal assumptions about the relationship between social activity and loneliness?
2. What are your objectives for the planned activities?
3. Is there variety in the activities offered?
4. To what extent do activities promote opportunities for self-determination and feelings of personal control?
5. What barriers exist that discourage lonely tenants from social involvement or participation?

Personality and Preferences for Social Involvement

Each tenant brings with her values and beliefs regarding socializing both within and outside the complex, needs for affiliation, temperament, social skills, and reasons for moving to senior housing. Overall, these personalities and life histories contribute to the social climate, level of social activity, and tenants' involvement with others. Tenants with low levels of social activity prior to moving to senior housing are more likely to experience isolation following their move (Carp, 1987). In contrast, sociable tenants are more likely to benefit from social activities offered. As a rule of thumb, if tenants evidence only patterns of stability or decline in activity level, there is a need to rethink existing social programs. If, on the other hand, there are tenants whose activity levels increase, decrease, and remain the same, chances are that the social programs are working (Cranz, 1987).

Housing managers must accept individual differences in social activity and preference for social activity among elderly tenants. What housing managers need to realize is that most older persons are satisfied with their current levels of social activity. Particular attention should, therefore, focus on tenants who are unhappy, lonely, or dissatisfied with their levels of social involvement. For these tenants, *innovative* social programming may reduce loneliness and isolation.

The following case study illustrates one elderly tenant's experiences with loneliness:

Mr. J

Mr. J, an 83-year-old widower, reports that he has not gotten over his wife's death, which occurred just prior to his move to senior housing 12 years ago. His only family contact is with several nieces whom he contacts by phone "just to have someone to talk to." Other family members are a brother and a stepson. According to Mr. J, he has not had contact with his stepson lately and his brother is "bothered" by Mr. J's phone calls. When Mr. J noted that he has difficulty remembering certain names, such as the President of the United States, he explained that he doesn't get the opportunity to talk to anyone, so he has "difficulty in calling this to mind."

To overcome Mr. J's problems with loneliness, a social service outreach worker arranged for a friendly visitor for Mr. J. The friendly visitor helps Mr. J with his shopping. Mr. J takes great delight in describing the difficult time he has had "training" his visitor to shop correctly. The bond between Mr. J and his visitor is apparent in the affectionate way that Mr. J describes their interactions.

Thinking about your tenants who experience moderate to severe problems with loneliness, answer the following questions:

How are the feelings of loneliness expressed?

What barriers prevent lonely tenants from reaching out to others for social interaction and support?

What actions have you taken to reduce feelings of alienation and loneliness?

SOCIALLY ISOLATED TENANTS

Adjustment to senior housing is affected by the older person's previous patterns of social participation. Socially isolated tenants have difficulty in adjusting to life in senior housing. There are two groups of isolated elders: lifelong isolates and those who have become isolated due to aging-related losses. Approaches to working with these two groups are different.

Lifelong Isolates

Lifelong isolates have experienced prolonged social isolation throughout their lives. They are socially disadvantaged when expected to adjust to the social life of communal living. Difficulties in adjusting are understandable because isolated elders have lacked a social arena in which to practice their social skills. Over the years isolates have missed opportunities for exercising social skills and learning skills for adjusting to new situations. As a result, they may fail to understand the consequences of socially inappropriate behavior.

With progressive social isolation, older persons suffer additional losses in their social abilities and experience increased risk for interpersonal problems. An explanation of how social isolation affects adjustment to group living is the "isolation-desocialization syndrome" (Bennett, 1973). The following describes this process:

> An old person in the community becomes isolated, then desocialized; he enters a home for the aged or some other setting, misperceives the norms and blunders socially soon after entry; others single him out, perhaps as a "troublemaker" and avoid him. He then becomes resentful and alienated, and finally he deviates further from the norms by becoming involved in overt conflict with staff members and/or other residents. (Bennett, 1973, p. 186)

Adjustment to the social norms of the housing complex depends upon a number of factors: (a) motivation to remain in the housing, (b) clarity of formal and informal norms concerning appropriate behavior, and (c) understanding of consequences when norms or rules are violated. Housing managers can assist isolated elders by providing clear information about the formal and informal norms of the complex and positive reinforcements for socially appropriate behavior.

Later Life Isolates

For others isolation is a recent phenomenon. Age-related losses, such as widowhood, declining health, or death of friends and family members result in progressive social isolation if older persons are unable to compensate for these losses (Rathbone-McCuan & Hashimi, 1982). As a consequence, isolated elders experience lowered morale, inability to cope with future losses, and loss of social skills. The threat of social isolation for certain groups of elderly persons is particularly great. For example, elderly women who have built their entire social lives around their spouse are particularly susceptible to social isolation when their spouse dies (Rathbone-McCuan & Hashimi, 1982; Sheehan & Mahoney, 1984).

Mrs. P

Mrs. P is 79 years of age. She has been a widow for the past 2 months. Prior to her husband's death Mrs. P had cared for her husband for 6 years until 2 years ago when she was unable to care for him. According to Mrs. P, her entire life was oriented toward providing care to her husband, at first caring for him at home and then visiting him daily at the convalescent home. Mrs. P is fortunate because she has an extensive informal support network. While she participates in a number of organized social activities, she noted, "Now I'm here by myself and I find it very lonesome."

The move to elderly housing for some older persons is an event that can lead to social isolation. Tenants who have moved from another community to be near an adult son or daughter may be particularly vulnerable if the move disrupts old, irreplaceable social relationships with friends and neighbors.

For tenants with well-developed social skills and outgoing personalities, the move to senior housing offers exciting opportunities for making new friends.

Poor health, poverty, and ageist attitudes are other potentially isolating events. Poor health and severe functional impairment leave tenants unable to actively participate with other tenants. Limited financial resources may also prevent social participation with other tenants. If social activities are costly, such as eating out, planned excursions, movies, or other events, poor tenants experience very real barriers to their social participation. Finally, older persons who hold negative attitudes toward old age may avoid interactions with other tenants because they do not want to associate with those "old people." Such ageist attitudes prevent full social participation in senior housing. If a tenant lacks social skills to initiate new social involvements then isolation will result.

Housing managers can assist later life isolates by providing:

- Support, encouragement, and reinforcement of efforts to exercise their social skills
- Opportunities to engage in both one-on-one and group activities

- Linkages to other tenants with similar interests
- A positive social climate that creates an environment in which tenants feel comfortable participating in social activities with one another

FOSTERING A POSITIVE SOCIAL CLIMATE IN SENIOR HOUSING

Housing managers who seek to foster a positive social climate in their senior housing complex should thoughtfully consider what elements of the housing environment can be changed or modified to improve the quality of life for elderly residents. Specific consideration should focus on the (a) management policies, (b) services and resources, (c) tenant and staff characteristics, and (d) the physical environment. (Chapter 5 discusses the impact of design and the physical environment on tenant well-being and quality of life.)

Management Policies

Management policies have a tremendous impact on the social climate, quality of life of elderly residents, opportunities for social interactions, and resident satisfaction. In fact management policies are more important than the physical environment for promoting tenant interaction and satisfaction (Cranz, 1987; Pynoos, 1987). Policies that promote resident autonomy and self-determination increase significantly social participation and involvement among elderly tenants (Pynoos, 1987; Rodin, Timko, & Harris, 1985; Timko & Moos, 1990). In contrast, restrictive policies destroy tenant well-being and opportunities for social interaction. As Pynoos (1987) relates, restrictive management policies have been linked to "depression, a sense of helplessness, and accelerated decline" (p. 33).

Policies that promote resident autonomy and independence, however, inevitably involve "costs" that housing managers should understand. Policies that promote autonomy result in an inevitable tension between autonomy and support (Feingold & Werby, 1990). Among the costs or conflicts that can arise in response to policies that promote independence are decreased "efficiency" of the organization and conflict with staff's perceptions. First, policies that promote resident self-determination involve tension between the efficiency of the organization and tenants' rights for self-determination. Management policies must strike a reasonable balance between resident autonomy and the smooth functioning of the housing complex (Pynoos, 1987). Second, staff members may experience conflicts when a resident's choice is perceived as less than ideal or involving potential risk to the tenant. Actions that enable tenants to exercise their right of self-determination can cause conflict between staff members' self-image as caring persons and elder's right to choose. Despite these tradeoffs, the value of policies that promote independence versus "taking care of" cannot be diminished (Feingold & Werby, 1990).

Policies that encourage tenants to participate in setting rules and influencing decisions contribute to increased tenant satisfaction and a sense of pride and ownership among elderly tenants (Pynoos, 1987). Structures such as active tenant organizations and meaningful social programming build a sense of community among elderly tenants and increase social interaction. Finally, management policies help to give tenants a sense of direction, set realistic boundaries concerning the rights and responsibilities of elderly tenants, increase mutual support among tenants, and reduce the likelihood of interpersonal conflicts (Timko & Moos, 1990).

When the actions of management and staff are not consistent with stated policies inevitable conflicts will occur. Recent experience at a senior housing complex underscores the importance of management's **actions** toward elderly tenants.

The stated policies of the senior housing complex are to maximize tenant involvement and self-determination; however, on a recent visit to the complex, we experienced a situation that clearly failed to support tenants' needs for self-determination.

Office hours for the complex were listed on the door (10:00 to 12:00). When we arrived at 10:00, the Office door was locked. Sounds from within the Office indicated that several staff members were present. However, a knock on the door produced no response. Five minutes later, a second, much louder knock produced a voice from within saying that the Office was not yet open. By 10:15, a final knock resulted in the door being opened. Not surprisingly, subsequent interviews with several tenants who live in this complex noted that tenants felt remarkably little influence in shaping or influencing decisions at the complex.

Housing managers and staff must be keenly aware that policies are not enough. For elderly tenants in senior housing, *actions speak louder than words.*

Planned Activities and Resources

Planned social activities and resources are an integral part of senior housing. Carefully chosen social activities can achieve a number of different goals: (a) create a sense of community among elderly tenants, (b) establish linkages between elderly tenants and the broader community, (c) utilize the personal resources of tenants by providing volunteer activities to serve frail tenants or less fortunate members of the community (e.g., disadvantaged children, frail elderly, etc.), (d) promote opportunities for mutually supportive relationships, (e) stimulate opportunities for social interaction and making friends, (f) bring together generations to increase mutual awareness and understanding, (g) provide enrichment activities that promote personal growth and development, (h) offer opportunities for fun and entertainment, and (i) enhance cognitive and intellectual ability and reduce egocentrism among elderly tenants (Cohen, Bearison, & Muller, 1987). Programming efforts should encompass a variety of activities because older persons, just like younger persons, have different needs and desires for social activity. Activities should include on-site activities, activities involving the broader community, and activities that include family members. Creative activity planning should include educational/information programs, social get togethers, community service volunteer programs, and fun/entertainment.

Activities should consider the impact of limitations in health, mobility, or economic resources on tenants' ability to participate in certain activities. Activities should not be oriented solely to a specific group of elderly tenants, such as healthy, functionally independent elders or more affluent seniors who can afford the costs associated with certain activities. Activities should include opportunities for both group activities and one-on-one activities. Many tenants may be uncomfortable in group activities and prefer opportunities for social interaction that involve one other person. What housing managers fail to realize is that, despite differences in content, most, if not all, activities they offer are group activities.

Read the list of social activities (Table 6.1). Is this program available in your housing complex? If yes, what are your goals for the program? How effectively does this activity accomplish its stated goal? For each activity, who are the tenants who attend? Does your housing offer a variety of different types of activities (e.g., group versus one-on-one, on-site versus off-site, closed versus open to the broader community, etc.)? What additional activities do you feel should be incorporated into your housing?

Implementation of a single program can have a number of benefits to program participants, community, and society. For example, a volunteer telephone reassurance program for latch key children offers multiple benefits. Elderly volunteers experience opportunities to help children and their families by providing a valued service, promotion of self-esteem, and opportunities for social interaction. Benefits to the community include breaking down misperceptions between younger persons and older adults, developing channels of communication between children and the elderly, and providing a needed service to families. Finally, recognition of the continuing contributions of older persons breaks down societal stereotypes that perceive the elderly as useless, unproductive, or a burden on society. Working to dispel negative attitudes about aging and old people will inevitably change how older tenants perceive themselves and how they define themselves in relation to the housing complex, the community, and society.

Aggregate Staff and Tenant Characteristics

Both staff and tenant characteristics contribute to the social climate in senior housing. Staff characteristics include size, background and training, personal qualities, and turnover rate.

Opportunities for ongoing in-service education should provide staff with critical knowledge and skills for working with at risk and impaired elderly tenants. Conflicts between promoting resident autonomy and self-determination and staff's desire to "help" elderly tenants must be dealt with on a regular basis. Well-intentioned,

TABLE 6.1 Social Activities in Senior Housing

Resident Committees	*Visitation Programs*
Tenant Council	Friendly Visitors
Newcomers Committee	Telephone Reassurance
Care and Share Committee	High School Visitors

Social Activities	*Volunteer Programs*
Monthly Potluck Supper	Tutoring Program
Weekly Coffee Klatch	Latch Key Children
Bingo, cards, etc.	Senior Advocates
Brown bag luncheons	

Education/Information Program	*Crafts/Hobbies*
Contemporary Events/Issues	Sewing, quilting, etc.
World Affairs	Woodworking
Information about community programs	Gardening
Arts	

Health Promotion	*Fun/Entertainment*
Exercise	Movies
Nutrition information	Fashion shows
Blood pressure screening	Talent shows

Personal Growth	
Life review, reminiscence	
Relaxation	

but overly helpful, staff increase tenants' dependence on staff members.

Staffing patterns should be as flexible as possible to guard against institutionalizing a need for a particular staff position. When a supportive service program is introduced, ongoing evaluation is essential. Phasing out a staff position dedicated to a particular program or reallocation of staff time is a sign of a successful program. Overall, housing managers need to identify creative ways to promote resident independence rather than promoting dependence to justify the need for more staff. While few senior housing complexes could be considered to have too many staff, a high staff-resident ratio reduces opportunities for tenant self-determination and influence (Timko & Moos, 1990). The linkage between size of staff and quality of life is important to consider.

Tenant characteristics that influence the social climate include heterogeneity among tenants, health and functional ability, and social resources. Differences among tenants decrease levels of social interaction and integration. As with people of any age, elderly persons select friends and acquaintances who are similar in age, socioeconomic status, marital and parental status, and general interests. As a rule, greater similarity among older persons increases levels of social interaction. The move to senior housing, however, may lessen the influence of certain factors on friendship formation. For example, marital status is less influential in the friendship formations of women in senior housing than in the community at large (Adams, 1985-1986). Efforts to increase understanding of the commonalities among residents can reduce the effects of "selection" factors by which potential friends are eliminated. Functional impairment may also inhibit social integration among tenants. The existence of the "poor dear" hierarchy decreases opportunities for social integration as frail tenants remove themselves from interactions to avoid the stigma associated with their frail condition.

Tenants' social resources influence the nature of their social involvement. Elderly tenants with greater social resources are more likely to engage in social interaction and take advantage of structures, such as Resident Councils, to exert influence on the housing complex. Housing managers and staff should be aware that in working with less socially advantaged tenants greater time and attention is needed to encourage and support involvement in the social life of the complex. Activities, program structures, and planned social opportunities must be modified to respond to the special needs and abilities of different tenant groups. Flexible programming is particularly important in being able to respond to the needs of elderly tenants as they age in place.

For housing managers, ongoing attention to the role of management policies, planned activities and resources, staff and tenant characteristics, and the physical environment is essential for sincere efforts to build a positive social climate within senior housing.

WHAT HOUSING MANAGERS CAN DO
TO INFLUENCE THE SOCIAL ENVIRONMENT

Throughout this chapter suggestions have been offered concerning just what housing managers can do to positively influence the social environment in senior housing.

From your very first encounter with a prospective tenant, your actions, demeanor, and attitude set the tone for the older person's perception of the housing environment. Being warm and friendly, not overly intrusive, conveys your sincere interest in the older person. Enthusiastically describing the opportunities for social involvement and social participation in the housing complex establishes a positive orientation to the social benefits of senior housing. The description of social opportunities should be realistic. Don't create unrealistic expectations about the opportunities available.

Be sensitive to the older person's concerns about the move. How does the move to senior housing affect the older person's ability to maintain previous friendships and relationships? What feelings and attitudes are expressed concerning social relationships during the initial interview? Are there particular interests expressed by the prospective tenant at this time?

Be aware of the important position that you occupy in many elderly tenants' social worlds. For many, you are seen as a friend, someone who can be counted on in times of emergency (Wolfsen et al., 1990). It is important always to treat elderly tenants with respect and guard against betraying the relationship. Work to reduce ageist attitudes within yourself, tenants, and the community. Be constantly vigilant to avoid manifestation of the "poor dear" hierarchy in your own actions and the actions of others.

Be attuned to changes in the social climate in your housing. Prompt attention to social problems will forestall problems from becoming even more intense. Review your rules and regulations to determine their effect on the social environment in your housing. Use both formal and informal contacts with tenants to identify potential and real problems that exist for your tenants. Provide appropriate forums to address emerging issues. Offer or sponsor educational/informational programs to increase interpersonal awareness and sensitivity and breakdown existing barriers that prevent full participation by all tenants. Regularly review the activities offered at your complex. Encourage the involvement of community groups with elderly tenants to break down barriers and increase understanding of senior housing.

Finally, your thoughts and actions should always focus on building social linkages between elderly tenants and others. Help tenants to exercise social skills and learn new social skills to handle future situations. Avoid situations that promote dependency among elderly tenants. Define your role as that of helping tenants to take care of themselves.

GUIDELINES FOR HOUSING MANAGERS IN PROMOTING A POSITIVE SOCIAL ENVIRONMENT

1. Recognize and accept the heterogeneity among elderly tenants.
2. Respect individual rights for autonomy and self-determination.
3. Facilitate planned activities that promote social growth, social support, and social competence among elderly tenants.
4. Encourage activities that promote autonomy and feelings of self-determination among tenants.
5. Be a role model demonstrating respect and social concern for tenants.
6. Promote socially supportive linkages among elderly tenants, elderly tenants and their families, and elderly tenants and community social service providers.
7. Provide opportunities for the broader community to be involved in activities in your senior housing complex.
8. Maximize the choices among various types of activities available to tenants.
9. Avoid situations that promote dependency among elderly tenants by encouraging the exercise and development of social skills.
10. Never betray the trust and confidence of your elderly tenants.

7

Social Support in the Lives of Elderly Tenants

Having others with whom we share our lives, our secrets, and even our everyday tasks, not only improves our psychological well-being, but also improves our health and increases our chances for survival. For people of any age the prescription for good health is to be socially involved with others and exercise your relationships. Whether a person is 20, 40, or 75 years of age, the importance of supportive relationships cannot be overestimated.

This chapter examines social support in the lives of elderly tenants and strategies to foster and strengthen social support. Among the specific issues examined are:

- What is meant by social support?
- Who are vulnerable or "at risk" tenants?
- Is all assistance that tenants receive beneficial?
- How important is family support in tenants' lives?

The remainder of the chapter examines roles for housing managers and social service providers in mobilizing support for elderly tenants.

WHAT IS SOCIAL SUPPORT?

Social support refers to interactions with others that provide help or assistance. Assistance may be in the form of instrumental help (e.g., help with housework, financial aid, transportation, help during times of illness, personal care, such as bathing, grooming, etc.), emotional support (e.g., love, kindness, caring, etc.), information (advice, financial counseling, information about services, etc.), and affirmation or positive regard (respect, acceptance, validation, etc.). Although just how social support contributes to better health is unclear, support received by older persons helps them in dealing with stress and stressful life events.

HOW DO ELDERLY TENANTS RECEIVE SUPPORT?

Older persons receive support through their *social networks.* The social network consists of all those people who are available to (but do not necessarily) provide support or assistance (Antonucci, 1990). Potential members of an elderly tenant's social network include: spouse, adult children, siblings, nieces, nephews, cousins, friends, neighbors, clergy, physicians, health care professionals, social service providers, and paid helpers. Social networks vary widely in both size and composition. At one extreme, isolated elders have no one upon whom they can rely. At the other extreme, some older persons have very large social networks.

Two case studies of senior housing residents illustrate the concept of social network.

Mrs. J, age 83, is a widow. She has lived in senior housing for the past 10 years. She has four adult children—three sons and one daughter. She has no contact with two of her three sons. She has regular contact with her remaining son and only daughter. Of Mrs. J's seven brothers and sisters, only two sisters are currently alive. Mrs. J, however, has lost contact with one of her two surviving sisters. All Mrs. J's close friends have died. She has limited contact with one neighbor who drops by to check on her every few days. Mrs. J continues her involvement in St. Mary's Church, where she has been an active member. She receives no community services.

Figure 7.1 depicts Mrs. J's social network. Members of Mrs. J's network who provide support are: a son and daughter, one sister, a neighbor, and her church. Network members who could potentially provide support are Mrs. J's two sons, a sister, and community service providers. The lines in the diagram connecting Mrs. J to the people in her social network reflect those relationships that involve the exchange of assistance.

The size of an older person's network, however, is not a guarantee that needed assistance will be received. While large networks increase the likelihood that help will be provided, size is less important to an older person's well-being than the quality of the support. If network members misperceive an older person's assistance needs, they will provide help that is either ineffective or detrimental or no help. Overly attentive or anxious family members who provide "too much" help deprive older persons of opportunities for personal growth. This "smother love" promotes unnecessary dependence and reduces feelings of self-determination. In other instances, good intentioned but "overly helpful" social service providers deprive tenants of their right to self-determination.

The second case study describes the social network of Mr. B (Figure 7.2).

Mr. B is 84 years old. Mr. B never married and has led a somewhat isolated life. Of his three siblings, only a younger sister has survived. Mr. B, however, has lost contact with her. Mr. B, due to severe arthritis, is confined to his apartment. A paid homemaker through the local VNA provides 2 hours of assistance to Mr. B every 2 weeks. The manager of the complex in which Mr. B lives either drops by or phones Mr. B every week to make sure he is all right. Mr. B does not participate in any organizations or groups.

Mr. B's only surviving family member is a sister. While potentially a source of support, the fact that he has lost contact with her makes this unlikely. The size of Mr. B's network makes him vulnerable to nursing home placement if his health or functional ability declines.

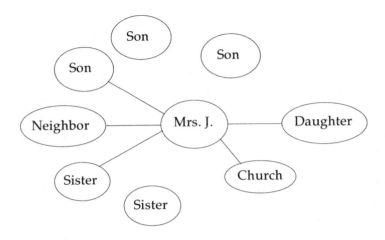

Figure 7.1.

IS ALL ASSISTANCE THAT ELDERLY
TENANTS RECEIVE BENEFICIAL?

We know from our daily lives that not all interactions with others positively influence well-being. Repeated negative interactions devastate an older person's well-being. In fact, negative interactions exert a stronger influence on psychological well-being than positive interactions (Rook, 1984). The self-esteem of elderly tenants who are functionally impaired and unable to care for themselves is particularly susceptible to the negative effects of excessive help. Negative interactions interfere with an impaired older person's ability to maintain the illusion of competence in interactions with others (Taylor & Brown, 1988). Without sources of positive interaction, elderly tenants with disabilities may come to define themselves as incompetent, dependent, or worthless. An important question for anyone concerned about the quality of life for older persons is, "To what extent do interactions with others promote tenants' feelings of competence, self-worth and personal dignity?"

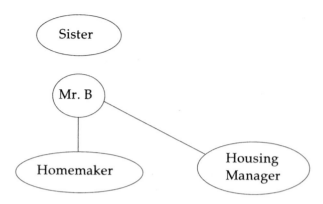

Figure 7.2.

WHO ARE VULNERABLE OR
"AT RISK" ELDERLY TENANTS?

Tenants with limited or nonexistent social networks are vulnerable when changes in health, functional ability, or other stressful events occur. Vulnerable elderly include elderly without family and tenants who rely on a single caregiver. Because families are the single, most important source of assistance older persons receive, tenants without family experience significant disruptions when their health declines or other losses occur. The elderly without families are particularly vulnerable when health problems occur. During short-term illness, they either turn to friends or do without help. When long-term chronic illness occurs, however, elderly without family experience a significant threat of institutional placement.

For tenants who rely on a single caregiver, the viability of the support system is threatened if the health of the caregiver deteriorates, if the caregiver is no longer available through death, relocation, or other responsibilities, or if the caregiver experiences emotional exhaustion or burnout.

Housing managers and social service providers should assist these "at risk" tenants to create, expand, or strengthen their social networks. Untapped sources of support include neighbors, friends, church groups, or formal community-based service agencies.

WHAT HAPPENS TO SOCIAL NETWORKS WITH AGING?

As people age, changes occur in their social networks. Changes include: losses or gains in network members; altered relationships between the older person and network members; changing relationships among network members; changes in the frequency and types of services provided; and overall changes in the composition of the network. From a systems perspective, the components of the network are interrelated. The death of a close friend, termination of a homemaker service, or a daughter's move to another city, are examples of changes that impact on the entire support system. In part, the disruption brought about by such changes depends upon the centrality of the absent person in providing assistance.

The entire support system consists of three subsystems—informal (family, friends, and neighbors); formal (governmental and volunteer agencies that provide services); and quasi-formal (organizations that tie the person to the broader community). Each subsystem possesses a unique set of characteristics that has an impact on the way support is delivered. Ideally these subsystems work together to meet elderly tenants' needs. This, however, is not the typical situation. Rather, the majority of older persons rely exclusively on support provided by family, friends, and neighbors (Manton & Liu, 1984).

INFORMAL SUPPORT FROM FAMILY, FRIENDS, AND NEIGHBORS

Help provided by family, friends, and neighbors is termed informal support. It is both the preferred source of assistance and the most common type of help that older persons receive. Estimates indicate that approximately three quarters of community-living elders rely exclusively on informal support, while only 5% rely solely on paid support (Manton & Liu, 1984).

One of the most important features of informal support is its flexibility in responding to older persons' needs. Unlike community service programs that involve eligibility requirements and other restrictions, the informal system responds personally to the needs of the older person.

How Important Is Family Support in the Lives of Frail Elderly Tenants

Discussions about later life families inevitably illicit strong emotions about what later life families do, what they should do, and how important families are to older persons' well-being. Take some time to reflect on your own attitudes and how these attitudes influence your work with families.

To what extent are older persons isolated or abandoned by their families?

How important are families to the well-being of older persons?

How do your attitudes about families affect your ability to work effectively with tenants' families?

What problems do you find difficult in your work with families?

A review of the gerontological literature provides interesting and somewhat paradoxical findings concerning families: First, **CONTRARY TO POPULAR BELIEF, OLDER PERSONS ARE NOT ISOLATED FROM OR ABANDONED BY THEIR FAMILIES.** In fact the overwhelming majority of older persons report frequent contact with family. Frequent contact, however, is not related to better psychological well-being. For some families, frequent contact is motivated by feelings of guilt, obligation, or indebtedness to an elderly relative rather than affection. In other instances, frequent contact is associated with increased health problems in an elderly relative's life.

Second, **FAMILIES PROVIDE THE OVERWHELMING MAJORITY OF CARE THAT FRAIL ELDERLY RECEIVE.** Family support is the critical factor that enables frail older persons to remain living in the community. Families are particularly helpful in providing help when an older person is ill and in providing assistance with activities such as shopping and transportation. Families are also the preferred source of care, particularly during times of illness. Few families, however, are prepared to provide for the long-term chronic care needs of dependent older persons. Over time, as an elderly relative's care needs increase, many caregivers experience a wide range of negative consequences: frustration, anger, guilt, physical and emotional exhaustion, loss of privacy, and deterioration of their own health (Brody, 1985).

Third, **DESPITE THE BURDENS OF PROVIDING CARE, FAMILIES ARE RELUCTANT TO REACH OUT FOR HELP FROM OUTSIDE AGENCIES.** Both institutional and personal factors interfere with families seeking help from community service agencies. Institutional barriers include: (a) restrictive eligibility requirements, (b) costly services, (c) bureaucratic red tape, (d) impersonal services, (e) fragmentation of services, and (f) lack of available services (Hooyman, 1983). Personal barriers include: (a) lack of knowledge about services, (b) values that stress independence and self-reliance, and (c) fear of seeking help. Other personal barriers to seeking help outside the family are feeling guilty about transferring responsibility, perceptions that providers do not understand their personal situations, view of providers as not really "caring" about the older person, and fear or mistrust of "strangers" in the home (Springer & Brubaker, 1984).

Finally, **LATER LIFE FAMILIES, LIKE FAMILIES OF ANY AGE, BRING WITH THEM A RANGE OF EMOTIONS, FEARS, INSECURITIES, AND UNRESOLVED INTERPERSONAL CONFLICTS.** Some adult children, unable to deal with their parent's declining health, gradually withdraw from visiting their elderly parent because it is too painful to watch them fail. In other cases adult children overprotect elderly parents due to feelings of guilt, fear of losing a loved parent, or fears of their own aging (Kuypers & Bengston, 1983). In still other instances, families abandon responsibility for frail, dependent relatives because they have unrealistic expectations about what senior housing can do. They assume that the housing manager will provide for all their parent's needs. Other families bring with them a lifelong history of unresolved interpersonal problems. In these families, as the dependencies of the parent increase, the intensity of the interpersonal problems also increases.

Working With Later Life Families

In working with families, housing managers and social service providers should:

- Recognize the diversity that characterizes later life families and get to know families
- Plan activities to involve families in the life of the complex to strengthen the ties between older persons and their families
- Recognize families' needs for support

Realistic expectations about what families can and cannot do rest upon understanding the strengths and weaknesses of each family. Take advantage of opportunities to get to know families and for families to get to know you.

The Needs of Families Caring for Impaired Elderly Tenants

Most families are unprepared to deal with the complex problems that occur as older persons experience multiple chronic health problems. As a result, families have increased support needs that frequently go unmet. Their support needs include: emotional support, information, and instrumental assistance.

Emotional Support

Simply listening to a caregiver's concerns and feelings in a nonjudgmental way provides an opportunity for family members to express their often conflicting feelings. Further, reinforcing the positive aspects of the family's behavior provides positive feedback for family caregivers. Helping a family member understand how much her visits mean to an elderly tenant reinforces this behavior and strengthens the family's commitment to caring. Providing family members with information about community-based family caregiver support groups may help family members receive additional support.

Information

Families need clear cut information about the housing, their relatives' needs, and community services. As part of the management role, housing managers have several tools to respond to these informational needs. First, clear residential policies help families to define their role in providing support and to understand the limitations of the housing in accommodating excess levels of frailty. Use of the Personal Care Sponsor Statement is a useful tool to help families understand the importance of their involvement. Other tools include a Handbook for Personal Care Sponsors and a Directory of Community Services (See Chapter 4). Accurate information about aging, functional health, compensations in the face of disability, and community services helps family members to perceive accurately an older person's need for support and access needed support services. If families feel assisted in their efforts to provide care, they can cope more effectively with the day-to-day demands of care.

Instrumental Assistance

If frail tenants rely on assistance from several different sources, the demands on the family are lessened. Sources of help outside the family include: community-based support services, help from friends and neighbors, care from physicians and other health professionals, help from clergy and church-based organizations, and assistance from volunteer organizations. Expanding the number of persons in vulnerable tenants' support networks provides relief to families by sharing responsibility for essential support tasks.

On-site planned services and activities can be implemented to overcome some of the barriers that prevent families from seeking needed help. Examples of activities include:

- On-site services to reduce the impersonal nature of the formal service bureaucracy
- Community service fairs to bring service providers into the housing to increase knowledge about services and decrease fear of the unknown

- Innovative service-delivery model programs that enable residents to pay for services on a sliding scale
- Volunteer advocacy programs to assist elderly tenants with entitlements, paper work, and so on

Efforts should be made to avoid situations that overly burden a single caregiver. Because vulnerable elderly tenants' ability to continue living in the community depends upon the availability of informal support, housing managers should be constantly aware of the potential burdens that a single primary caregiver faces. A "burned out" primary caregiver is unable to provide any assistance to a vulnerable tenant. In planning and implementing these and other types of programs, housing managers assume a set of new roles and responsibilities. These new roles include advocate, coordinator, linker, and facilitator. These new roles are discussed later in this chapter.

GUIDELINES FOR WORKING WITH FAMILIES

1. Recognize and accept the diversity among later life families.
2. Get to know tenants' families and encourage families to get to know you.
3. Develop procedures for addressing the informational needs of older families.
4. Assist families in dealing with their feelings.
5. Provide opportunities for family caregivers to express their concerns.
6. Actively listen to families' concerns.
7. Help families understand the importance of the support they provide.
8. Help families in accessing help from community service providers, friends, neighbors, and so on.
9. Implement specific activities/programs that overcome the barriers that prevent families from reaching out for help.
10. Avoid overburdening a single caregiver involvement.
11. Help families accept the new reality of their situation.
12. Recognize and respond to the family's needs for support.
13. Help the family set realistic goals and expectations.
14. Involve families in the social life of the housing community.

Friends and Neighbors in the Lives of Elderly Tenants

Friends and neighbors are part of the informal support system. There are, however, important differences in the support functions that friends and neighbors perform. These differences are often overlooked because the term "friendship" is inappropriately used to refer to a wide range of social relationships (e.g., acquaintances, colleagues, and causal encounters). However, for purposes of discussion, we use the term "friendship" in a much more restrictive sense.

What Is So Special About Friendship?

According to gerontologists, friends are "good medicine." We all know how important it is to have a friend. Having a friend means knowing that there is at least one person who knows us, cares about us, desires to spend time with us, and with whom we share aspects of our life. Knowing that we have a friend makes us feel valuable to at least one other human being. Friendship reflects an intimate knowledge of another person, shared history, common backgrounds, common interests and experiences that have fused together a strong emotional bond. Friendships are a source of emotional support, affection, companionship, and help with everyday tasks. For many tenants, however, the ability to maintain long-term friendships is limited when health problems arise. Loss of long-term friends through death or relocation is particularly painful for older persons. The ability to make new friends depends upon a number of factors: the social climate in the complex, the person's social skills and personality, opportunities for social involvement, and his or her desire for friends.

Housing managers can facilitate friendship formation among tenants by:

- Providing a social climate that encourages neighborly interaction and support
- Offering a range of both group and one-on-one activities within the complex
- Linking tenants with similar interests and backgrounds

How Much Do Neighbors Help One Another?

Living in close proximity, neighbors are in an ideal position to help one another. Proximity, however, does not guarantee that neighbors will become friends or that neighbors will provide help to one another. In fact, when elderly tenants name their "friends," few cite tenants who live in their complex. Further, even when high levels of social interaction occur, relationships with other tenants are generally considered as less important and less emotionally close than other relationships.

Interventions aimed at strengthening informal support among neighbors must recognize tenants' feelings toward their neighbors. The following excerpts from interviews with senior housing tenants provide insight into some of these feelings (Sheehan & Mahoney, 1984). Reasons for limited social involvement with others in the complex were: (a) desire to avoid conflict, (b) frailty, (c) limited financial resources, (d) loss of previous friendships, (e) reluctance to ask for help, and (f) perceived discrimination.

Desire to Avoid Conflict. Mr. B, an 84-year-old widower, noted that while he is "friendly" with other tenants, he keeps his distance to avoid his "gossipy" neighbors. He would rather be by himself than be involved in all the "talk" about neighbors.

Frailty. An 82-year-old widow, badly crippled by arthritis, Mrs. C said, "I talk to everybody and the people are nice enough . . . but to be a real, real friend I can't be . . . I can't especially now go anywhere . . . But before when I could go, I went on a few trips before, but now I can't." Home-bound, Mrs. C has not received any help from her neighbors since she was hospitalized 4 months ago.

Limited Financial Resources. Mrs. K cited financial reasons that limit her involvement with her neighbors. Mrs. K, who admitted that some months she must choose between eating and buying her prescriptions, noted that she is embarrassed to have her neighbors visit in her home because she has such old, dilapidated furniture.

Loss of Previous Friendships. Mrs. A, age 79, reported that she had friends when she moved to the senior housing complex 9 years ago. Over the years, however, several friends have gone to convalescent homes and one has died. Presently, her only social involvement is limited contact with her next door neighbor and a "telephone friend" from the complex who occasionally phones her. She described herself as "very lonely" and admitted that she is being treated for depression. Mrs. R, age 82, misses her "special friend" who moved to another housing complex. Although active in a number of social activities, she does not have a neighbor with whom she shares a special friendship. In fact, she does not have any emotionally close relationships with her neighbors.

Reluctance to Ask for Help. Reluctance to ask for help is expressed by tenants who do not want to be a "bother to anyone." In the words of Mrs. D, an 83-year-old widow, "I don't bother with them. . . . I'd rather be by myself, not to be a bother."

Perceived Discrimination. Some tenants discriminate against certain racial or ethnic groups, while others discriminate against frail or impaired tenants. Discrimination can range from avoidance to open hostility. Efforts to keep wheelchair-bound tenants away from public view is an example of discrimination.

What Can Housing Managers Do to Facilitate Neighborly Support?

Efforts to encourage mutual support, if done appropriately, offer invaluable opportunities for increased emotional and instrumental support. First and foremost, housing managers' efforts to establish a positive social climate set the stage for enhancing neighborly support. In developing interventions, particular attention should be directed to avoid situations that encourage "helping" that deprives tenants of feelings of self-determination or results in either excessive help or unwanted help. Possible activities or programs that housing managers can initiate include:

1. *A Volunteer Credit Bank:* Recognizing the need for tenants to exercise their right of self-determination and desire to avoid unbalanced relationships, housing managers can establish a "Volunteer Credit Bank." The volunteer bank operates on the principles of a bank. Older persons make deposits into their account (credits for

volunteer activities to other tenants). In the future when the volunteer needs services, she can draw upon her account. "Support" that is received has been "earned" by previous volunteer efforts.

2. *Sensitivity Training:* Housing managers may offer programs designed to increase tenants' sensitivity and awareness of older persons with special needs. As part of programming designed to promote personal growth and effectiveness, sensitivity programs could address special issues such as physical disabilities, developmental disabilities, and dealing with emotions. Trained professionals could be asked to develop such programs to increase sensitivity and decrease the barriers among elderly tenants.

3. *Helping Tenants Understand the Multiple Opportunities for Providing Support:* One of the barriers that prevents tenants from helping one another is a narrow conception about what "support" or "help" actually means (Sheehan, 1988b). As tenants age, they may be unable or reluctant to take on responsibility for helping frail tenants with instrumental tasks, for example, transportation, housekeeping, cooking. Programmatic structures, such as Resident Councils, and Care and Share Committees, can help tenants define alternative means for providing neighborly support. For example, a telephone reassurance program for homebound elderly tenants provides volunteers an opportunity for responding to frail tenants' needs. Telephone partners may link together two very frail neighbors, each of whom is providing a much needed service.

FORMAL SUPPORTIVE SERVICES

Community services and entitlement programs make up the formal support system. Formal services include both entitlement and direct service programs. These programs include: Social Security, Supplemental Security Income, Medicare, Medicaid, adult day care, homemakers, home health aides, visiting nurse, counseling, friendly visitors, companions, chore services, energy assistance, home-delivered meals, respite care, legal services, case management, home repair, weatherization, personal care services, senior centers, employment programs, volunteer programs, outreach, shopping assistance, transportation, escort services, telephone reassurance, and congregate meals. For most programs only a small fraction of eligible older persons receive assistance. Chapter 8 examines the formal service network available to provide supportive services to elderly tenants.

QUASI-FORMAL SUPPORT

The final component of the support system is assistance available from the quasi-formal support system—religious, fraternal, ethnic, and neighborhood organizations—that connect the person to the larger society. For older persons membership in these organizations provides a sense of belonging and connectedness. Unlike the impersonal formal system, churches, fraternal organizations, or ethnic associations provide assistance on the basis of a personal tie that exists between the individual and the group. Given the meaning and centrality of these organizations in older persons' lives, older persons may be more accepting of help provided by these groups (Hooyman, 1983). Quasi-formal organizations are an overlooked resource for elderly tenants. Churches and religious organizations with a long tradition of responding to human need are an outstanding source of assistance for elderly tenants (Sheehan, 1987).

Housing managers and social service providers can assist tenants in accessing quasi-formal support and advocating for needed services. Advocacy efforts should include: (a) identification of unmet need among tenants, (b) efforts to bring existing services into the complex, and (c) mobilization of quasi-formal organizations to develop new services to meet the needs.

NEW ROLES FOR HOUSING MANAGERS
AND SOCIAL SERVICE PROVIDERS

The previous discussion of barriers that prevent the full mobilization of the helping network for frail older persons calls for the identification of a new set of possible roles—empowerer, advocate, coordinator, facilitator, developer, linker, and resource provider— for housing managers and social service providers (Biegel, Shore, & Gordon, 1984). Overall, the goals for these new roles are to overcome barriers that prevent the full mobilization of the support systems serving vulnerable elderly tenants and to strengthen the support systems serving elderly tenants. Although there is some overlap in the activities associated with each role, it is helpful to discuss each activity separately to illustrate the range of options available to housing managers and social service providers.

Empowerer

Housing managers and social service providers empower elderly tenants when they encourage, support, and facilitate tenants' rights for personal control and self-determination. Actions that empower elderly tenants include: (a) implementation of residential policies and structures that maximize tenant involvement in decision making, (b) provision of information concerning existing community services and entitlement programs, (c) reinforcement of positive social interaction and social skills, (d) respect for the dignity and the privacy of the individual, and (e) provision of educational and personal growth programs for tenants.

Advocate

Advocacy efforts on behalf of elderly tenants seek to obtain needed services and resources. Advocacy efforts include bringing community services on-site to better serve vulnerable elderly tenants, encouraging formal and quasi-formal support organizations to develop needed services, working on community councils on aging to represent the needs of elderly tenants, and networking with social service and health professionals to acquire knowledge about services for elderly tenants.

Coordinator

Given the fragmentation of the formal support system, housing managers and social service providers can direct their efforts to bring together existing services to provide a more comprehensive base of services for elderly tenants. Networking among housing, social service, and health care professionals can help to reduce some of the fragmentation that characterizes the formal support system. Efforts to identify "gap filling" community services serving frail elderly tenants also come under this role.

Facilitator

Any activity that seeks to expedite older persons receiving needed services is part of this role. Examples of activities that fall under this role include: facilitation of resident structures such as Resident Councils, Care and Share Committees; informational programming; community services informational fairs; and offering space to community service programs serving the elderly.

Initiator/Developer

Housing managers and social service providers who have identified an unmet need among elderly tenants can function to develop supportive service programs for tenants. Program development should be viewed as a way of creatively responding to unmet needs among tenants. Funding for demonstration or model projects may be available from area foundations, area agencies on aging, or local business sponsors.

Linker/Intrasystem

Housing managers may work to bring together elements of the informal system (family, friends, and neighbors) to serve the needs of elderly tenants more effectively. The interventions previously described for strengthening support from family, friends, and neighbors fall under this role.

Linker/Intersystem

Ideally the formal, informal, and quasi-formal support systems work together to provide needed assistance; however, because in most cases this situation does not occur, professionals may assume responsibility for coordinating between subsystems of the support system to more effectively serve elderly tenants.

Direct Service Provider

In some cases housing managers provide direct services, counseling, and other resources to elderly tenants. As Care Managers for tenants who lack other sources of support, housing managers may find themselves providing limited direct services to isolated tenants.

Resource Provider

One of the most important functions that housing managers perform is providing information about services, entitlements, and other sources of support to elderly tenants. To enact this role, housing managers must learn about all the potential sources of support available to elderly tenants.

8

Formal Services in Senior Housing

As elderly tenants age in place, the importance of formal services increases. Formal services such as home care, transportation, home-delivered meals, home nursing services, and home health aides can provide essential supportive services that enable elderly tenants to avoid unnecessary or premature institutional placement. In most cases use of formal services can either supplement or complement the support that elderly tenants receive from family, friends, and neighbors. In the case of isolated elderly with disabilities, however, many rely exclusively on formal services because they lack other sources of support (Tobin & Toseland, 1990).

As more and more tenants experience moderate to severe limitations in their ability to care for themselves, housing managers, social service providers, and health care providers need to be knowledgeable about the array of formal supportive services to assist elderly tenants to live independently in the community. This chapter examines the various types of formal services available to meet elderly tenants' needs. Particular attention focuses on the role of the housing manager in helping tenants access needed services.

FORMAL SERVICES

The formal service system consists of a wide range of service-delivery agencies that provide different types of assistance. Agencies that provide services to older persons exclusively are part of the "aging network" that has emerged in response to the perceived needs of growing numbers of elderly persons. Programs and services that make up the aging network include homemaker agencies, home care agencies, elderly transportation systems, nutrition programs, Meals on Wheels, home repair and handyman programs, legal assistance programs, health care entitlement programs, income-transfer programs, friendly companion programs, long-term care institutions, volunteer programs, job banks and job training programs, elderly outreach programs, adult protective services, adult day care, respite programs, case management, and senior centers.

Other services that make up the formal service system are generic, nonelderly services, including: counseling programs through community mental health centers, alcohol and drug treatment programs, local social service agencies, support groups, food stamps, services to the blind, and so on.

Together aging network and generic formal services make up the formal service system available to older tenants.

NATURE OF THE FORMAL SERVICE SYSTEM SERVING ELDERLY TENANTS

The "formal service system" does not represent a single system. Services are fragmented and lack a central or unifying structure. These services represent a "patchwork" or "band-aid" approach to meeting the needs of an increasingly heterogeneous elderly population (Tobin & Toseland, 1990).

The nature of the service-delivery system creates obstacles for those who attempt to access services—older persons, families, housing professionals, and social service professionals—including: different eligibility requirements, lack of integration both within and between aging and generic services, and territorial issues that keep service agencies from cooperating. First, because services are provided by a wide range of different agencies, access to or eligibility for services is based upon different criteria. Agencies operate under different program guidelines that specify the clients to be served, type and duration of benefits, and geographic region served. Formal services, unlike services provided by family or friends, provide assistance only to persons who meet eligibility requirements. For example, some programs only serve low-income older persons; others are available only if prescribed by a doctor; still others are available only for a certain period of time; while some are available only to persons who live in a specific geographic area.

Second, the lack of integration both within the aging network and between the aging and generic service network (services outside the aging network) hinders efforts to develop a comprehensive package of services for elderly persons with disabilities. Many social service professionals in the aging network are unfamiliar with services available from the DD/MR, mental health, or other nonaging networks. Similarly, service professionals working outside the aging network are unfamiliar with the range of aging-based services. Opportunities for developing comprehensive services are lost due to lack of knowledge and understanding concerning the full range of service alternatives available in the community. In other instances, duplication or overlapping services between the aging and generic service networks creates confusion among housing professionals concerning the most appropriate community resource to meet elderly tenants' needs for information and/or services.

Finally, in some communities territorial issues prevent full cooperation among the range of helping professionals potentially available to assist elderly tenants. Sources of tension and conflict around territorial issues can arise from philosophical differences concerning the most effective way to meet elderly persons' needs, efforts to justify the need for a particular agency or service when duplication exists, and political pressures on service agencies to serve the largest number of clients possible. As housing managers attempt to work with the formal service system, they inevitably confront an uncoordinated, complex service-delivery system.

For most programs only a small fraction of eligible older persons receive services. The challenge for housing managers and social service providers is to link elderly tenants with needed services.

NECESSARY SKILLS FOR HOUSING MANAGERS AND SOCIAL SERVICE PROVIDERS

The reality of the fragmented service-delivery system makes it imperative for housing managers and social service providers to be:

- knowledgeable about the full range of services available
- skillful in referring elderly tenants to appropriate services
- creative in implementing new roles to assist tenants in receiving needed services

The following case studies of elderly tenants illustrate a range of different formal service configurations to maintain vulnerable elders in their own apartments.

Mr. A, age 84, has lived in senior housing for the past 15 years. He suffers from multiple chronic health problems that severely limit his ability to live independently. Through the provision of both community-based and in-home services, Mr. A is able to continue living in his home. A critical component of the formal services that Mr. A receives is provided by a local adult day-care center he attends 3 days a week. The center provides him with opportunities for social contact and socialization with his "buddies." The center also provides medical supervision and access to proper nutrition. In addition to the community-based service provided through the adult day-care center, Mr. A receives the services of a home health aide 2 days a week. The provision of essential services that enable Mr. A to age in place, in part, accounts for his remarkably optimistic outlook on life.

Mrs. L, age 89, relies solely on in-home services. Mrs. L has been homebound for the past year due to her severe arthritis. She has extreme difficulty in carrying out several critical activities of daily living such as preparing her meals, maintaining her apartment, and bathing. While Mrs. L's only daughter does her weekly grocery shopping, Mrs. L also receives the services of a homemaker, friendly visitor, and a home health aide. Without the formal services that Mrs. L receives, she would be unable to remain in senior housing. Prior to receiving formal services, Mrs. L was feeling increasingly depressed and lonely due to her progressive social isolation.

Mrs. M, age 79, has suffered recurrent episodes of depression throughout her life. After the death of her husband, 9 months ago, Mrs. M felt that she no longer wanted to live. The intensity of her depressive symptoms increased over time. With the encouragement of the housing manager, Mrs. M sought medical treatment for her depression. Under a physician's care, Mrs. M attends a psychiatric day-care center 2 days a week. As a result of medication and the therapeutic services of the adult day care center, Mrs. M's depressive symptoms have disappeared.

As each of these case studies suggests, solutions or strategies for meeting the service needs of vulnerable elderly encompass a range of different services. For elderly tenants with needs for social, psychological, and physical assistance, complex configurations of formal services can enable them to age in place with dignity and independence.

The first step for housing managers and social service providers in linking elderly tenants with services is to recognize the possibilities and constraints that characterize the formal service system. Second, housing managers should participate actively and interact with local social service and health care professionals to understand programs and advocate for needed services. Housing managers should take advantage of opportunities to serve on local boards of community agencies in the aging and nonaging service networks to better understand the service delivery system in their city, town, or region. (Chapter 11 provides some suggested activities for housing managers to network with other professionals to assist elderly tenants with disabilities.)

The ability to get to know the resources in a given community, in part, depends upon the size of the community (Roff & Atherton, 1989). In small communities professionals can easily learn information about formal services. In much larger communities learning about formal services is a much more strenuous endeavor. In these communities professionals may rely on existing agencies that provide information about community services. These information and referral programs are designed to help people locate needed community services. In many communities information and referral agencies have prepared a resource guide that lists community services. The information provides a valuable resource for getting to know services in a particular community or region. Because, however, the information contained in most printed materials becomes obsolete rather quickly, information should be personally verified to be useful to housing professionals and social service and health care professionals.

The next step is to develop a Personal Resource Guide that supplements, complements, and updates information available from the resource guide (Roff & Atherton, 1989). The Personal Resource Guide lists all services available to tenants in senior housing. Each entry in the resource guide should identify: the name, address, and telephone number of the agency; the type(s) of services available; restrictions or eligibility requirements for receiving services; and benefits. The guide should also identify helpful key staff persons and their areas of expertise. This information can be developed only through interactions with the professionals who make up the helping network.

Information about key agency personnel is particularly important when providing information to elderly tenants. Because not all professionals are equally helpful or accessible to older persons, whenever possible, referrals should assist elderly tenants to reach an empathetic, patient, and responsive ear. A single contact with a cold, disinterested, bureaucratically minded service professional can abruptly end the help-seeking behavior of an elderly tenant.

Mrs. M, age 83, with the encouragement of her family, neighbors, and the housing manager, has acknowledged a need for a companion to assist her several days a week; however, Mrs. M is unsure where to find such assistance. The housing manager suggested that she call her State Department on Aging. When she made the call, Mrs. M talked to a worker who sounded totally uninterested in Mrs. M's situation explaining that there was no program available through the Department on Aging. The worker then suggested that she could call her local area agency on aging, local commission on aging, or two or three home heath care agencies. Following this initial request for help, Mrs. M was frustrated and confused concerning what to do next.

If Mrs. M decides to call one of these agencies, do you think she will get the help she needs? Do you think Mrs. M will decide it is too much hassle to locate the service and give up? How many phone calls do you think Mrs. M will make before her help seeking behavior is extinguished by the bureaucratic formal system? While Mrs. M's response to seeking help cannot be generalized to all elderly tenants, it is safe to assume that many tenants seeking help either get lost or discouraged in their efforts to receive services.

A suggested format for entries listed in the Personal Resource Guide follows:

Personal Resource Guide

Agency: _____

Address:_____

Telephone:_____

Names of Key Staff Members:

_____

_____

Names of Helpful Staff Members:

_____

_____

Type of Services Provided:

_____

_____

Eligibility Requirements/Restrictions on Services:

_____

_____

Special Information About Agency:

_____

_____

_____

Information contained in a Personal Resource Guide should be revised regularly to reflect current changes such as those in staff turnover, changing eligibility requirements, helpfulness or effectiveness of the service delivery agency. If possible, data contained in the Personal Resource Guide should be computerized to make updating the guide easy.

FORMAL SERVICES FOR ELDERLY TENANTS WITH DISABILITIES

Goals of Formal Services

The overall goal of services for older persons should be to promote the autonomy and self-determination of the client. The more specific goals of services should consider the functional level of the older person. For older persons who are relatively independent and free from major functional limitations, services should prevent deterioration of abilities and enhance well-being. For elderly tenants whose functional abilities are moderately impaired, services should enhance their functioning, strengthen and support the efforts of caregivers, and restore lost functioning, whenever possible. Finally, for elderly tenants who are severely impaired, services should prevent unnecessary institutionalization and provide appropriate institutional care when needed (Tobin & Toseland, 1990).

Types of Services

Various systems have been proposed to categorize services available to older persons (Tobin & Toseland, 1990). For purposes of discussion, the following categories are used to describe services: in-home services, health services, care/case management, financial/legal assistance services, transportation and escort, and information and referral.

Many formal services that enable elderly tenants to live in the community are funded by the Older Americans Act. These services are available under the auspices of Area Agencies on Aging (AAAs). Information about the location of the AAA serving your region is available by calling your State Unit on Aging.

Area Agencies on Aging serve as a focal point in their region to bring together a range of service providers and community groups that serve the needs of older persons. Area Agencies on Aging identify the needs of older persons in their region and mobilize resources to respond to those needs. While few provide direct services to older persons, they are an extremely valuable resource for information about programs and services available to older persons.

Services funded by AAAs include information and referral, homemaker/home health aides, chore services, congregate and home-delivered meals, transportation, and other supportive services. Area Agencies have funded a variety of innovative service programs targeted specifically to meeting the needs of elderly tenants in senior housing.

In-Home Social Services

In-home social services include homemaker, home maintenance and chore services, emergency response systems, home repair, homemaker, in-home assessment, Meals on Wheels, outreach, shopping assistance, and telephone reassurance. Several of these in-home services particularly beneficial to elderly tenants who have aged in place are discussed briefly.

Homemaking, Home Maintenance, and Chore Services. Homemaking, home maintenance, and chore services provide invaluable assistance to maintain elderly tenants in their apartments. Homemaker services for tenants with disabilities are particularly important in helping elderly tenants meet the conditions of their lease. Among the services available are light housekeeping, shopping, laundry, errands, meal preparation, home maintenance, heavy cleaning, and yard work. As elderly tenants' ability to carry out various instrumental activities of daily living deteriorate, the services of a homemaker may be critical to support their ability to perform essential activities for living in independent housing.

Meals on Wheels. Meals on Wheels delivers hot, nutritious meals to older persons who are homebound or unable to prepare their own meals. The meals are delivered by volunteers 5 days a week. Because meal preparation and eating are critical ability areas that directly impact on an elderly tenant's ability to live in independent senior housing, Meals on Wheels provides a supportive service that can make the difference in whether or not an elderly tenant can maintain herself in senior housing.

Telephone Reassurance. Telephone reassurance programs provide a telephone check in service to provide a sense of security to elderly tenants who live alone. The program involves a daily phone call at a predetermined time made by the elderly tenants to a central office or a phone call made by a volunteer to the elderly tenant. If there is no answer, family, neighbors, or police are notified to check on the welfare of the elderly person. For homebound, isolated elderly tenants, the services of a telephone reassurance program can dramatically increase their feelings of security.

Friendly Visitor Program. Friendly Visitor Programs provide volunteer visits to lonely, isolated older persons. The volunteer visits the elderly tenant once or twice a week to provide companionship. The volunteer also gives a helping hand with personal or household problems. Friendly visitors provide companionship, help with errands, or just someone to listen to their concerns.

Friendly visitor programs may be available through local churches, social service agencies, and other agencies within the community.

Health Services

A second category of services for elderly tenants involves a wide range of health services. These include: in-home health and personal care, adult day care, Alzheimer's day care, Alzheimer's evaluation centers, geriatric assessment units, health screening programs, home health aides, home health nursing, hospice programs, and rehabilitation services.

In-Home Health and Personal Care. Home health agencies provide supervised personnel to respond to older persons' health care needs. Health services include help with taking medications, changing dressings, and other skilled nursing services. Personal care services for persons needing help with activities of daily living such as bathing, grooming, and dressing are also provided to older persons who require these services.

Adult Day-Care Programs. Adult day-care programs provide social and recreational programs and medical services for elderly persons with disabilities. Day-care programs are particularly appropriate for older persons who need help with self-care activities or require some supervision. Socially isolated tenants with unmet personal care needs may find adult day care particularly beneficial. Activities and opportunities for social interaction provided by adult day-care centers provide social stimulation for isolated elderly tenants. An assessment performed by the staff of an adult day-care center can develop a service plan to meet the individual needs of an elderly tenant.

Day-care programs typically operate 5 days a week. Hours vary but most are in operation from 9 a.m. to 5 p.m. Centers are under the auspices of hospitals; long-term care facilities; and religious, fraternal, and other nonprofit agencies. The services provided at adult day-care programs vary. Most provide limited medical supervision. This includes administration of medications and minor treatment. A registered nurse supervises this aspect of the program. Some programs involve a rehabilitation component. The services of a speech and hearing therapist, physical therapist, or occupational therapist may be available.

Adult day care can be available on either a long-term or short-term basis. For tenants in need of assistance with personal care who lack assistance from family or friends, adult day care provides an alternative for delaying or preventing institutional placement.

Some adult day-care programs specialize in providing care to Alzheimer's patients. Information about adult day-care programs in the local area can be obtained from either the area agency on aging or state unit on aging.

Care or Case Management Services

A third category of services involves care or case management services. Case management agencies, however, do not provide direct services. The services offered by case management agencies include consultation, assessment service, coordination/monitoring service, and comprehensive care management. After assessing the older person, case management service agencies take responsibility for developing a care plan and monitoring the services that are delivered. The care manager selects the best services to meet the older person's needs. The care management agency contracts with local service providers to secure necessary services for clients.

Transportation and Escort Services

Transportation services, which help older persons get around in the community, are provided to doctors' offices and other medical services, community facilities, shopping, and other services. Transportation may be provided by a senior citizen van or under a contract with a local taxi company to provide transportation at a discount rate. Older Americans funds are used to purchase or lease a van and pay for the driver's salary.

Transportation services, which enable elderly tenants to maintain their independence, are particularly important in geographic regions that lack public transportation. Escort services are provided in some communities to assist older persons in getting around or shopping.

The Older Americans Act provides funds for transportation and escort programs in local communities.

Information and Referral (I & R) Services

Information and referral agencies provide information about where to go for help. I & R services provide older persons, their caregivers, and concerned professionals with access to telephone information about services available in a local community to meet specific needs such as energy assistance, Medicaid, Medicare, Social Security, and other areas of concern to elderly persons.

Information and referral programs frequently publish informational brochures that list information about community resources. A recent demonstration Information and Referral Program initiated in the New England region provides a "hot line" for information requests.

Legal Services

Legal services are designed to protect the rights and interests of older persons. The specific functions that legal services play include protecting the welfare of older persons, securing entitlements, safeguarding their property, and providing advice and counsel concerning financial and business affairs. Basic legal issues that elderly persons may confront include income maintenance programs (Social Security, Supplemental Security Income, general assistance, Veterans' benefits, private pensions, food stamps); health care (Medicare, Medicaid, Veterans' benefits); consumer affairs; employment discrimination; tax relief; property transfers (wills, trusts, living wills, probate); and protective services (conservatorship, guardian, power of attorney) (Spring & Kuehn, 1990).

The importance of legal assistance to secure access to benefits has increased since the beginning of the Reagan years. In the face of increasing pressures toward cost containment, many benefit programs designed to serve the elderly have become increasingly adversarial (Spring & Kuehn, 1990). Therefore older persons must increasingly depend on legal services to assure access to benefits to which they are entitled.

Check with your Area Agency on Aging to identify advocacy groups that provide assistance to older persons to secure benefits and entitlements.

Power of Attorney. Power of Attorney involves a legal procedure enabling an older person to give an "attorney-in-fact" authority to act on his or her behalf. Power of Attorney authorizes the "attorney-in-fact" to handle the older person's bills, real estate and banking transactions, and legal affairs. The Power of Attorney lasts only as long as the person is mentally competent. If the person becomes no longer competent, the Power of Attorney is no longer valid.

Durable Power of Attorney. In some states older persons may specify a power of attorney that continues even if the older person becomes incompetent. Durable power of attorney authorizes the older person's representative to handle all financial and legal affairs involving the older person. Because states treat durable power of attorney differently, housing managers and social service providers should determine the relevance of this legal procedure in their state.

Guardianship. If an older person is judged by the court to be mentally incompetent, a guardian or conservator is appointed by the court. The guardian is responsible for decisions involving the elderly person's legal affairs, medical decisions, and so on.

Living Wills. Living wills provide a statement concerning an older person's wishes concerning the use of life-sustaining procedures. The Living Will enables an older person to state his or her wishes in advance. Various states have enacted statutes concerning Living Wills.

Tenants' Rights. Tenants must be advised concerning their legal rights and right to appeal. As previously discussed, elderly tenants need to be informed of their rights involved in applying to the housing, their rental rights and obligations concerning continued tenancy and eviction, and rights and channels of appeal. Legal services, the Bar Association, or State Unit on Aging provide information about lawyers specializing in tenants' rights.

Protective Services

Protective Service Programs are designed to protect the rights of older persons who are being abused or neglected. Protective services may be called in to investigate situations in which an older person who lives alone is not physically or mentally competent to care for himself or herself. In other cases protective services may investigate suspected abuse of an elderly person.

Protective services programs intervene in cases where an older person is suffering physical, mental, or emotional abuse or neglect.

In Connecticut the Protective Services Units of the Department of Human Resources assume responsibility for protecting elderly persons from abuse, neglect, exploitation, and abandonment. Under state law, social workers, medical professionals, police, clergy, and nursing home staff who believe that an older person is being abused or neglected must report the situation to a regional ombudsman of the Department on Aging. If the elderly person is being neglected or abused, a social worker from the Department of Human Resources develops a comprehensive plan to address unmet needs. Protective service workers will intervene immediately if the person's health or safety is in imminent danger. If the older person refuses services and is judged mentally competent, services cannot be provided. If the older person is determined to be mentally incompetent and in danger, Protective Services, through probate court, will seek the appointment of a conservator.

Making a Referral

As professionals seek to assist elderly tenants in accessing formal services, they should follow guidelines to ensure that all interventions foster independence and self-determination even among the most impaired elderly tenants. In their book, *Isolated Elders*, Rathbone-McCuan and Hashimi (1982) describe guidelines for maximizing older persons' involvement in solving their own problems. According to these guidelines, it is critical that interactions with elderly tenants are not geared to "do something" for them. Efforts to "do something" for elderly tenants promote dependency and result in missed opportunities for tenants to learn new problem-solving skills. Even the most impaired elderly tenants should be actively involved in providing input into the intervention process. Contacts with elderly tenants should, rather, always focus on skill building and increasing tenants' ability to handle future situations.

In working with elderly tenants, the goal of interventions should be the development of a broader support system. This goal can be accomplished by:

1. Providing elderly tenants with information about social support available
2. Assisting elderly tenants to select the best possible source of support
3. Helping the tenant to develop skills to access the social support system
4. Encouraging elderly tenants to accept supportive services from a broad range of social supports (Rathbone-McCuan & Hashimi, 1982)

Housing managers and social service providers must help elderly tenants to build their skills. Specific attention should focus on how to use referral services, how to communicate effectively, and how to be more assertive in securing basic needs (Rathbone-McCuan & Hashimi, 1982). All intervention contacts with elderly tenants should assist tenants in more effectively utilizing existing resources and developing increased skills for gaining needed supports.

The process of assisting elderly tenants to identify and access needed services depends upon housing managers having sufficient information about both the elderly tenant—age, address, income, and prior contacts with other agencies—and the service agency—name of agency, telephone number, address, services provided, eligibility requirements, and cost (Perry, Kurland & Citron, 1989).

When making a referral it is important to follow a few specific suggestions to increase the effectiveness of the referral. Perry, Kurland, and Citron (1989) identify five basic rules for making referrals. These are:

1. Know necessary information about both tenant and agency ("Know your facts").
2. Be persistent ("Be prepared to sell your case").
3. Insist on getting the right answers ("Find out to whom you're speaking").
4. Network with social service personnel ("Build up a network of contacts").
5. Don't be discouraged when services may not appear to be immediately available ("Be creative"). (p. 157)

The reality is that the referral process is not as easy as it might first appear; however, being prepared to follow the suggested guidelines helps to reduce many of the barriers that prevent successful referrals. Housing managers who succeed in linking elderly tenants with services have responded creatively in building interpersonal and programmatic bridges between elderly tenants and the service network. Housing managers who have been unsuccessful in their efforts to link older persons and services, in part, have failed to do the necessary groundwork for successful referrals. In other instances housing managers may be unsuccessful because programs or services are not available.

As social service programs experience increased cutbacks that limit service availability, housing managers will find it more and more difficult to link elderly residents with existing services. Chapter 11 discusses innovative approaches to developing social service programs in senior housing when services are not readily available in the community.

Housing managers should never consider the formal support system in isolation from other sources of support or assistance in elderly tenants' lives. In their efforts to assist older persons in locating needed services, housing managers may find themselves assuming a new set of roles—coordinator, linker (both intrasystem and intersystem), facilitator, advocate, resource person—to foster elderly tenants' opportunities for personal growth and self-determination.

9

Special Mental Health Issues in Senior Housing

INCREASED attention has focused on a number of special mental health challenges that confront housing managers and social service providers in their work with elderly tenants. This chapter addresses some of these special challenges: alcoholism and substance abuse, cognitive impairment, and depression. Efforts to examine these issues systematically have been limited, because few researchers have studied how these problems present themselves in senior housing. Anecdotes from housing managers and others, however, report frightening stories about suicides, interpersonal conflicts, violence, and other problems. The following discussion, whenever possible, draws upon information derived from experiences in senior housing. In areas where limited information exists, the discussion relies on knowledge about these problems within the general aging population.

ALCOHOLISM AND SUBSTANCE ABUSE

Anecdotal information from housing managers suggests that substance dependence is a major problem among elderly tenants. According to these accounts, many of the falls, fires, and other accidents that occur in senior housing can be linked to excessive alcohol use among elderly tenants. While exact figures concerning the prevalence of alcohol abuse among elderly tenants are not available, Brody (1982) suggests that:

> One of their most distressing and persistent problems is alcoholism and alcohol abuse, which causes an inordinately high proportion of serious and nagging difficulties. The rates of alcohol associated fires, falls, starvation and neglect, and violence are simply not known, but increasingly whispered about in these communities for the elderly. (p. 125)

Failure to identify tenants in senior housing who suffer from alcoholism and alcohol-related problems can lead to serious problems. First, undetected alcohol abuse endangers the health and safety of the abuser. Second, unrecognized problems associated with substance abuse endanger the safety of other tenants. Finally, the failure to detect alcohol abuse reduces the likelihood that the problem can eventually be treated.

Detection of Alcoholism and Alcohol Abuse

There is widespread agreement that alcoholism among the elderly is frequently overlooked. Detection of the problem is complicated by a number of factors that prevents accurate identification. First, manifestations of alcohol abuse are frequently attributed to other factors. Because many of the behavioral manifestations of alcoholism mimic diseases such as dementia and depression, housing managers and social service providers frequently misinterpret signs or symptoms of alcohol abuse as due to other factors. Competing explanations include "aging," failing health, depression, or cognitive impairment.

> Mr. Green, age 78, has lived in the elderly housing complex for 8 years. For the past 5 years, he has been widowed. During the past year the housing manager has observed that Mr. Green's ability to get around the complex has deteriorated. When he walks, his feet shuffle along the walk. Frequently Mr. Green appears unsteady on his feet. Last winter Mr. Green fell several times outside his apartment.

When asked if he was experiencing any problems or difficulties by the housing manager, Mr. Green acknowledged that his arthritis seemed to be getting worse lately. He did not admit to experiencing any other problems.

A second factor that complicates early and accurate detection of alcohol abuse is the fact that most elderly experience multiple health problems (Tobias, Lippmann, Pary, Oropilla, & Embry, 1989). While Mr. Green's arthritis does limit his ability to get around, this is not the only reason for his mobility problems. His unsteady gait and recurrent history of falls are, in fact, due to his problem drinking. A third factor that complicates early detection is that the majority of elderly tenants live alone. Excessive drinking behind the closed doors of a tenant's apartment can go undetected for a very long time without anyone being aware that a problem exists. For tenants who have withdrawn from family, friends, and work, there are relatively few occasions when others may become aware that a problem exists. Because the "independent" environment of senior housing enables tenants to remove themselves from interactions with others, progressive social isolation enables abusers to hide their alcoholism successfully for a long time.

To protect tenants' right to privacy, some managers may equate noninterference with ignoring problem behaviors. Then the early signs of abuse will go undetected (Tenant Assistance Program, 1991).

For those who are not isolated, family members may deny or refuse to acknowledge the existence of an alcohol-related problem; and, therefore, they shield the tenant from identification. A desire to protect an elderly relative or to avoid the stigma associated with alcoholism can be powerful motivators that prevent even those closest to the elderly tenant from acknowledging that a problem exists. Families of elderly women may be particularly reluctant to acknowledge that a problem exists.

Other factors that prevent detection include: (a) the tendency of housing managers and social service providers to deny that a problem exists or that the problem is severe enough to warrant intervention, (b) lack of knowledge concerning the signs or manifestations of alcohol abuse, (c) lack of knowledge about treatment alternatives, and (d) stereotypes and myths surrounding both aging and alcoholism. Previous failures to educate professionals concerning alcoholism among the elderly keep them from pursuing aggressively efforts to detect the problem.

As a result, elderly alcoholics are extremely successful in avoiding detection —making them and their problem "invisible" in senior housing, leading to missed opportunities for early intervention.

Early Detection of Alcohol Abuse

Early detection of problems involving alcohol and drug abuse among elderly tenants is a critical activity for housing managers. Managers cannot rely on signs of either acute intoxication or withdrawal to determine that a problem exists.

The signs or manifestations of alcoholism or alcohol abuse among the elderly are:

- frequent falls or staggering
- anxiety
- depression
- uncontrolled hypertension
- malnutrition
- confusion or fluctuating mental status
- diarrhea
- dyspepsia
- poor grooming or self-neglect
- general physical deterioration
- recurrent or unexplained injuries

Because early recognition and proper treatment can bring about recovery in 80% of those suffering from some types of addiction, housing managers aware of the signs or manifestations of abuse should encourage elderly tenants to seek treatment for their problem (Bauwens, 1986). Knowledgeable housing managers are in an ideal position to determine both the extent of alcohol abuse and alcohol-related problems among their residents.

Early detection and intervention are critical not only for the recovery of the elderly substance abusers, but also for the well-being of other tenants, management, and owners. According to John MacPhee of the Massachusetts Housing Finance Authority's TAP (Tenant Assistance Program, 1991), early intervention will result in "fewer accidents, flooding and fires, abuse and neglect of property, a reduction in lawsuits, fewer evictions, a reduction in security costs, fewer rents in arrears, lower turnover in management/staff" (pp. 1-2).

Types of Elderly Alcoholics: Early Onset and Late Onset

A useful distinction applied to alcoholism in the elderly is the difference between two categories of alcoholism: early-onset (before age 60) and late-onset (after 60). Early-onset alcoholism accounts for between 50% to 75% of elderly alcoholism (Atkinson, 1984; Bienenfeld, 1987; Gaitz & Baer, 1971; Tobias et al., 1989). Early-onset alcoholics are more likely to display unstable personalities and maladjustment. As a group, they are also more likely to have a family history of alcoholism (Tobias et al., 1989). As a general rule, their response to treatment is poorer than late-onset alcoholics.

The development of alcoholism after age 60 (late-onset alcoholism) has been linked to aging-related losses that older persons experience. Retirement, bereavement, health problems, separation, involuntary relocation, and family conflicts are some of the losses that may trigger problem drinking in late life (Morse, 1988). Although evidence linking a single stressful life event to late-onset alcoholism is inconclusive (Ekerdt, DeLabry, Glynn, & Davis, 1989), some older persons in response to devastating losses turn to alcohol as a means of coping with their loss or grief.

A recent study comparing early- and late-onset alcoholics seeking outpatient treatment for their addiction noted that the late-onset alcoholics were more likely to reside in senior housing complexes (Hurt, Finlayson, Morse, & Davis, 1988). The greater incidence of late-onset alcoholics in elderly housing is intriguing. One possible explanation is that previous aging-related losses, such as declining health, death of loved ones, and losses of friends and family, precipitated the move to elderly housing. As a result, their increased exposure to losses and later life stressors creates vulnerability that leads to the increased likelihood of developing alcoholism in later life.

Other possible explanations for the increased numbers of late-onset senior housing residents who seek treatment include: (a) the social milieu of senior housing, (b) the disruptive effects of the move to senior housing, and (c) the vigilance of housing managers in referring elderly alcoholics to treatment.

Housing managers and social service providers should be aware that the social atmosphere in some age-segregated housing complexes fosters the development of late-onset alcoholism for some tenants.

> Mr. G, age 74, moved into a posh retirement community, Burnham Towers, following the death of his wife. His social adjustment to community life was facilitated through the social contacts that he made during "happy hours" every afternoon at the complex. However, after a year, Mr. G referred himself to an outpatient alcohol treatment center. Prior to moving to retirement housing, Mr. G had never experienced any problems related to alcohol dependence. Early intervention led to a successful treatment outcome.

Second, for some elderly tenants who develop late-onset alcoholism, the move to senior housing may disrupt their previous social relationships. Feeling alone and isolated in their new environment some may turn to alcohol as a means of coping with feelings of isolation. Thus for some the move to senior housing may be a critical stressor that leads to increased susceptibility to alcohol abuse.

Finally, housing managers' attention to alcohol-related problems when they emerge may be a critical factor in assuring that late-onset alcoholics enter treatment programs. Whatever explanation accounts for these findings, there is no doubt regarding the importance of early detection and intervention to encourage tenants to receive needed treatment.

A third group of elderly problem drinkers has recently been identified—intermittent problem drinkers—who have experienced intermittent drinking problems throughout their lives (Pruzinsky, 1987). For this group as they experience aging-related changes, many of their primary motivations for controlling their drinking in the past (e.g., work, family responsibilities, etc.) are lost. If the social environment of senior housing puts few demands on tenants, many elders who have been intermittent drinkers throughout adulthood may begin drinking following their move to elderly housing.

The care and concern of housing managers and social service providers should be focused on making sure that elderly substance abusers receive the treatment they deserve. Because the prognosis is good for late-onset alcoholics when treatment is initiated (Tobias et al., 1989), housing managers should be strongly encouraged to identify alcohol-related problems in the early stages. Further, in an attempt to prevent alcohol-related problems from occurring, housing managers and social service providers should be sensitive to the impact of multiple stressors in the lives of elderly residents and the impact of the sociocultural milieu of senior housing (Amis, 1987; Brody, 1984) that can lead to the increased risk of developing late-onset alcoholism.

Feelings of Hopelessness and Helplessness and Alcoholism

Feelings of powerlessness, being unable to control the changes that are occurring in one's life, are particularly conducive to the development of alcoholism in later life (Osgood, 1987). For some elders who experience strong feelings of hopelessness and helplessness, there is a strong tendency to turn to alcohol as a means of coping. For these elders, persistent feelings that they are unable to exert any control over an unpredictable environment lead to the use of alcohol as an escape. As feelings of helplessness increase, alcohol abuse and thoughts of suicide may appear the only way of coping with a hostile world.

Social Isolation and Alcohol Abuse

For some elderly alcoholics, social isolation may be a key factor in the development of alcoholism in later life. It is, however, incorrect to assume that only the socially isolated elderly are at risk of alcoholism. While progressive social isolation may occur for some elderly abusers, as family and friends gradually remove themselves from interactions with the abuser, not all elderly alcoholics are isolated or abandoned by their families. In fact recent descriptions of elders seeking treatment for their addiction indicated that the majority were not socially isolated (Finlayson, 1984). The majority of elderly persons seeking treatment were described as "socially stable"—married and living with their spouse at the time of seeking treatment.

Consequences of Chronic Alcoholism

Alcoholism has serious consequences for the physical and mental health of elderly tenants. When alcoholism and problem drinking go untreated, tremendous social, emotional, and personal costs are incurred.

Among the adverse health problems that chronic elderly alcoholics experience are: cirrhosis, gastritis, gastrointestinal bleeding, hypoglycemia, alcoholic hepatitis, malnutrition, anemia, and pancreatitis. As a result, their ability to live independently is frequently at risk.

In addition to physical health problems, elderly chronic alcoholics experience increased incidence of psychiatric problems including dementia, depression, and even suicide. Estimates suggest that for about 10% of elders with dementia the cause is linked to their alcoholism. In other instances depression frequently coexists with alcoholism. For some depressed alcoholics the depression preceded their alcoholism (primary depression). Estimates suggest that approximately 10% to 15% of older persons suffering primary depression turn to alcohol as a means of dealing with their depression (Bienenfeld, 1987). In other cases depression results from problem drinking (secondary depression). The distinction between primary and secondary depression is important. If the person suffering from secondary depression becomes sober, chances are good that the depression will improve, but for elders who suffered depression prior to their alcoholism, abstinence does not relieve the depression. These elders will typically require antidepressants to manage their depression.

Suicide is also linked to chronic alcoholism. In the United States alcohol is linked to one third or one half of all suicides (Tobias et al., 1989). Among the elderly the link between alcohol and suicide is even stronger. In fact, this group is four to five times more likely to attempt suicide than the national average (Charatan, 1985). Housing managers should be particularly aware that depression and feelings of hopelessness are strongly related to the increased risk of suicide among elderly alcoholics (Beck, Steer, & McElroy, 1982).

Alcoholism is also associated with social costs and losses. Relationships with family, friends, and neighbors are either lost or become conflict-ridden in response to chronic alcoholism. During later life, when family support is so critical to the well-being of older persons, many chronic alcoholics find themselves alone with little support or assistance from family or friends. Lacking social support from family or friends, the chronic alcoholic is particularly vulnerable to institutionalization when health problems emerge.

Negative attitudes about aging and alcoholism held by family, friends, and professionals prevent positive actions to address the problem of alcoholism. Examples of negative attitudes that prevent referral to treatment programs include: "What else does he have to live for?," "Her drinking is all that's left for her. As long as she stays in her apartment, who is she hurting?"

When housing managers and social service providers recognize how barriers to identification operate in the lives of elderly tenants and their own lives, strategies for referring elderly abusers to treatment programs can be put into place. Because the prognosis for treatment for most elderly abusers is good and the personal, social and interpersonal costs of alcohol abuse are so great, it is unconscionable for professionals not to intervene to get elderly tenants the help they need.

ALCOHOL USE IN SENIOR HOUSING AND RETIREMENT COMMUNITIES

Some senior housing complexes may actually foster the development of alcohol-related problems among residents. If alcohol consumption is a strong part of the social life within the complex, then social norms and values within the complex can promote the development of problem-related drinking. In some affluent retirement communities, daily happy hours can create alcohol-dependence in elderly residents who have not experienced problems in the past. The extent to which "happy hours" and other social activities involving alcohol influences the development of problem drinking is unknown; however, the experiences of community-based alcoholism counselors provides evidence to indicate that for some late-onset alcoholics their problem is linked directly to the social environment. Managers of retirement communities should be aware that levels of alcohol consumption among their residents are significantly higher than those of other groups of older persons (Alexander & Duff, 1988). Further, levels of consumption are particularly high among gregarious, socially active tenants. Thus, according to Alexander and Duff (1988), for some retirement communities "drinking is part of the social interactive process" (p. 636).

The higher rates of alcohol consumption among retirement community residents may be due to both the continuation of previous life-style patterns of middle- and upper-middle class elderly who move to retirement communities (Alexander & Duff, 1988; Borgatta, Montgomery, & Borgatta, 1982) and the tendency of a significant group of residents to use drinking as a means of gaining social acceptance within the community.

Intervention With Elderly Alcohol Abusers

When problems associated with alcohol consumption occur, housing managers and social service providers need to be prepared to intervene. Adequate preparation to address the problem includes: (a) knowledge of the signs and symptoms of abuse, (b) attitudes of concern and availability to assist tenants, (c) realistic attitudes about aging and alcoholism that facilitate positive action, and (d) specific action strategies for intervention that protect the rights of the individual. Housing managers and social service providers should never ignore the problem.

The TAP Program of the Massachusetts Housing Finance Authority has developed a systematic program for housing managers to address alcoholism among elderly tenants (Tenant Assistance Program of the Massachusetts Housing Finance Agency, 1991). The program provides specific guidelines or steps for intervention with elderly tenants who suffer from alcohol abuse. The process involves the following five steps (Tenant Assistance Program of the Massachusetts Housing Finance Agency, 1991):

Step 1—Examine attitudes and prejudices that influence
management practice
Step 2—Set reasonable expectations
Step 3—Reality confrontation
Step 4—Accountability/Action
Step 5—Reprogramming with new messages

Step 1 involves the need for professionals to achieve understanding concerning their personal experiences with drinking and
negative attitudes and beliefs toward residents with drinking
problems. For professionals it is critical to understand how previous experiences with alcoholism affect their perceptions of the
problems among elderly tenants. In this step it is also extremely
important to understand how negative attitudes and beliefs can
influence the outcome of interventions.

Step 2 involves setting reasonable expectations for the role of
housing manager. Managers are not expected to function as alcohol counselors. This step involves defining "what you should,
could, would do for an elder resident who appears to be manifest-
ing a problem with alcohol" (Tenant Assistance Program of the
Massachusetts Housing Finance Agency, 1991, p. 3).

Step 3, Reality Confrontation, involves acknowledgment of alcohol abuse when it occurs. Housing managers should be aware
that, in some cases, what appears to be an alcohol-related problem
is not always the case. Reality confrontation involves expressions
of concern for the resident's well-being regarding the behaviors
observed. For the housing manager, reality confrontation involves
pointing out the problem behavior and expressing concern and a
willingness to help.

Reality confrontation also relates to efforts to prevent the development of alcohol-related problems among tenants. Housing managers need to encourage tenants to express their feelings associated with losses they have experienced. Meaningful social
programming and opportunities for elders to exercise autonomy
and control can be effective preventive measures for decreasing
vulnerability to alcohol abuse.

Step 4, Accountability/Action, involves both documentation of
problems when they occur and communication with the resident

concerning problem behavior. Housing managers need to be aware that by ignoring certain behaviors they permit or enable dysfunctional behavior to occur. When concerns arise concerning dysfunctional behavior, housing managers should not only document instances of the behavior, but also express their concern and availability, if needed. It is important to understand that "Managers do not have the 'right' to take action against a resident even when inappropriately using alcohol unless such abuse violates the conditions of the lease" (Tenant Assistance Program of the Massachusetts Housing Finance Agency, 1991, p. 4).

Step 5, Reprogramming With New Messages, involves providing factual information about alcoholism. To create a positive environment in responding to problems of alcohol abuse, the myths surrounding alcoholism must be replaced by information that "alcoholism is a disease; it is not an indicator of one's moral inferiority or one's lack of will power. Alcoholism is a treatable disease" (Tenant Assistance Program of the Massachusetts Housing Finance Agency, 1991, p. 5).

The following intervention strategy developed by the Tenant Assistance Program, Massachusetts Housing Finance Agency (1991, p. 6) provides concrete steps to follow to secure treatment for an elderly tenant.

See a Problem/Acknowledge It
A. Do this in privacy.
B. Be specific about what it is that you observed.
C. Be non-judgmental and a good listener.
D. Do not delay, act when you witness the behavior.
E. If the person is intoxicated, wait and talk with him/her when sober.
Suggest a Referral
A. Let person know you think it is useful for him/her to talk with someone knowledgeable about alcohol problems.
B. Explain your reasons; make it clear that you are concerned about their well-being.
Make a Referral
A. Decide who will call for an appointment - the resident or you.
B. Use a resource where you know an assessment for an alcohol problem is available.
Follow-Up
A. Make certain the call/appointment was made.

SOURCE: Tenant Assistance Program of the Massachusetts Housing Finance Agency, 1991, p. 6. Reprinted with permission.

Community Resources

In most states resources exist at the state and local level to support efforts to get elderly tenants into treatment. Frequently, however, there is little overlap or coordination between the alcohol treatment network and aging network (Rathbone-McCuan & Hashimi, 1982). Staff from alcohol treatment centers can provide invaluable information to housing managers on strategies for working with elderly tenants. Community-based treatment programs may also have developed specific programs for reaching elderly abusers. As part of their efforts, they may offer educational programs to increase older persons' awareness of the seriousness of the problem, the dangers involved in mixing drugs and alcohol, and community resources available to assist older persons with drug or alcohol dependence.

COGNITIVE IMPAIRMENT AMONG ELDERLY TENANTS

The growing numbers of cognitively impaired elderly residing in senior housing present a special challenge to housing managers and social service providers. Concerns about cognitively impaired tenants include: their diminished ability to care for themselves, confusion, wandering, threats to self and other tenants' safety, and fires and other accidents that damage the housing complex.

Work with cognitively impaired tenants is complicated by the many myths and stereotypes regarding the cognitive changes that occur with aging. Most pervasive is the belief that "senility" is a normal, inevitable part of growing old. At the outset it is important to point out: (a) that "senility" is *not* an inevitable consequence of getting old; (b) "senility," does not refer to a specific disease but rather refers to a wide range of cognitive and behavioral changes attributed to a variety of conditions; and (c) continued use of the term, "senility," is counterproductive to efforts to work with elderly tenants.

Mrs. T, age 87, has resided in Cromwell Gardens Senior Housing for 15 years. Lately she has increasingly expressed concerns about her forgetfulness and inability to concentrate. Several times during the past month she has complained to the housing manager about her growing difficulty in remembering things and inability to think clearly. The housing manager hearing Mrs. T's complaints assumed that at age 87 the cognitive changes that Mrs. T was experiencing were inevitable. She was becoming "senile." The housing manager, feeling that all she could do for Mrs. T was to provide reassurance and support, told Mrs. T that as we get older we all forget things.

This example illustrates how misperceptions and stereotypes about aging limit opportunities for successful intervention.

False assurances given to an older person that the cognitive changes that she is experiences are "normal" can have extremely negative consequences for the older adult.

For working with cognitively impaired elderly tenants, housing managers and social service providers need: (a) a basic understanding of the different types of conditions that result in cognitive impairment, (b) documentation concerning relevant changes occurring in an elderly tenant's cognitive functioning and behavior, and (c) effective strategies for working with cognitively impaired tenants.

Types of Cognitive Impairments

Many conditions that older persons experience are manifested by symptoms of cognitive decline, deterioration, or mental impairment. While some of these conditions are due to organic, irreversible changes in the brain that lead to inevitable loss of cognitive abilities, other conditions are due to extrinsic factors and can be treated. In the latter case, symptoms of cognitive decline can be reversed or eliminated. According to the National Institute on Aging, approximately 100 reversible conditions mimic irreversible dementing illnesses.

Conditions that mimic irreversible dementing illnesses include poor nutrition, adverse drug reactions, a minor head injury, and a high fever. Accurate diagnosis is critical because, if left untreated, many of these conditions can ultimately lead to permanent brain damage and sometimes death.

The primary distinction between the types of cognitive impairment is between organic (irreversible) and reversible causes of cognitive decline. The distinction is extremely important because the presence of cognitive symptoms of decline and deterioration does not always indicate an untreatable, irreversible disease.

Dementia: Irreversible, Degenerative Diseases

Dementia refers to a large number of irreversible, organic conditions that result in progressive intellectual decline and involve permanent damage to the brain. Dementia is not a single condition, but rather a group of dementing illnesses that have similar symptoms. Diagnosis of the presence of a dementing illness, such as Alzheimer's disease, is generally determined by ruling out the presence of other causes, such as depression, intoxication, infections, nutritional deficiencies, metabolic and endocrine disorders, and vascular diseases that mimic dementia. When an elderly tenant begins to experience significant deterioration of his or her cognitive abilities, such as extreme forgetfulness, difficulty concentrating, and severe memory loss, prompt action to secure a diagnosis is imperative to determine the underlying cause of the problem and proper course of treatment.

Diagnostic criteria for determining the presence of dementia or dementing illness include: loss of intellectual ability of sufficient severity to impair social/occupational functioning, memory loss, unimpaired consciousness, and presence or absence of organic factors. In addition, a person with dementia will demonstrate at least one of the following: impaired abstract thinking; impaired judgment; disturbances of higher cortical activity, such as aphasia (losses in using or understanding speech, apraxia (loss of ability to perform purposeful movements), or agnosia (deterioration of recognition/perception abilities); and personality change.

Dementia typically occurs late in life. It is extremely rare before age 50. With advancing age, the prevalence of dementia increases. The most common type of dementia is Alzheimer's disease, accounting for approximately 70% of all dementing illnesses. Other irreversible dementing illnesses include: multi-infarct dementia, Parkinson's disease, Pick's disease, Creutzfeldt-Jakob disease, and Huntington's disease.

The overall pattern of deterioration that accompanies dementia varies from person to person. For some the ability to perform very basic activities of daily living may be maintained, while in other cases this ability is lost even though the level of cognitive impairment is not as great. The rate of deterioration also varies across individuals. For some, cognitive deterioration occurs at an extremely rapid rate, while others live for many years with only slight deterioration of their cognitive abilities. In addition, there is great variation in the amount of time a person with a dementing illness lives following diagnosis. Estimates, however, indicate that, on the average, the person will survive 5 years following diagnosis. Despite individual differences in the course of dementia, certain changes occur as the illness progresses. In the early stage the older person has difficulty remembering recent past events. At this point the memory loss may be difficult to interpret. Memory lapses may be explained by normal forgetfulness, too much stress, or anxiety. If the individual begins to evidence strange or unusual behavior, the individual or family members propose a variety of explanations to account for the behavior. Over time, as cognitive decline progresses, the disease affects all aspects of the older person's behavior.

Diagnosis of Dementia. The importance of accurate diagnosis cannot be overstated. Accurate diagnosis depends upon a thorough physical, neurological, and psychiatric evaluation. Included in the evaluation are tests of mental status and specific tests, such as a brain scan. Only after such a thorough, comprehensive examination can an accurate diagnosis be made. If it is determined that the condition is curable, then a treatment program can be implemented. If it is determined that the older person suffers from one of the dementing illnesses, there is help to ease some of the symptoms. Medication can help relieve agitation, anxiety, and depression, and help in the case of insomnia. As part of the treatment program, care should be taken regarding proper nutrition and normalizing the daily routine of the older person.

Diagnosis should be conducted by a physician who specializes in geriatrics. The diagnostic process is so complex that it requires specialized training in geriatric medicine.

Alzheimer's Disease

The prevalence of Alzheimer's disease increases dramatically with advanced age. A recent study estimated that the prevalence rates for Alzheimer's disease increase from 3% for those 65 to 74 to 19% for those 75 to 84 years of age. Among the oldest old, persons 85 years of age and older, roughly 47% experience Alzheimer's disease with moderate to severe levels of impairment (Evans et al., 1989).

Given the dramatically "aging" tenant populations in many senior housing complexes, it would seem that dealing with tenants with Alzheimer's disease will be an increasing reality for housing, social service, and health care professionals.

Symptoms of Alzheimer's Disease. Alzheimer's disease is associated with gradual losses of cognitive functioning. As Cavanaugh (1990) states, among the symptoms that can occur with the disease are:

> declines in memory, learning, attention, and judgment; disorientation in time and space; difficulties in word finding and communication; declines in personal hygiene and self-care skills; inappropriate social behavior; and changes in personality (p. 305).

As the symptoms of the disease progress, the person increasingly may experience emotional problems. Among the most common emotional problems that coexist with the disease are depression, agitation, and paranoia.

Personality changes also occur with Alzheimer's disease. Some persons display aggressive behavior that can be very frightening. In the later stages of the disease, older persons may become increasingly passive and withdrawn. In the final stage, the deterioration has robbed the person of almost all abilities. The person in this extreme stage of decline has lost all verbal ability, the ability to walk, and the ability to control bowel and bladder functioning. As a result, the person is completely dependent on others for all basic care needs. An intriguing phenomenon noted by caregivers is "sundowning," whereby certain dementia symptoms are worse in the evening than in the morning (Cavanaugh, 1990).

As cognitive deterioration progresses inevitably, families and those close to the older person grieve over the loss of their loved ones, as all prior characteristics of the person are lost to the disease.

During the early stages of Alzheimer's, when memory loss is minimal, persons with the disease may have few difficulties coping with the demands of independent senior housing. Early signs of forgetfulness, such as forgetting where familiar objects are placed or forgetting previously well-known names, do not pose a serious problem. Elderly tenants may compensate for these memory declines by using strategies such as always keeping things in the same place or writing down important names to remember. For tenants who have lived in senior housing for many years, their familiarity with the environment helps them compensate for these initial losses.

As deterioration progresses, however, more troubling situations occur. Examples include getting lost while traveling to a familiar location, disorientation to time and place, aggressive or violent behavior, and inability for independent self-care.

Strategies for Working With Cognitively Impaired Elderly Tenants

Because diagnosis is critical, housing managers and social service providers can encourage and support cognitively impaired tenants to have their problem diagnosed. The first step in working with cognitively impaired tenants is the establishment of a trusting relationship between the elderly tenant and housing or social service professional. If such a relationship is established, tenants will be more likely to share their concerns about the changes that they are experiencing. Because the changes are frightening to older persons, many may deny that the changes are occurring. Often memory loss and other changes are attributed to "aging."

Allen (1986) has suggested that housing managers use "gentle persuasion" or an indirect approach when an elderly tenant shows signs of deterioration. Sincere concern expressed by the housing manager about the well-being of the elderly tenant may motivate the tenant to seek medical attention. Allen (1986) suggests, "You might tell a resident that you have noticed she is not as sociable as she once was and ask if she knows that many simple problems, like infections or a malfunctioning thyroid gland, can cause memory loss or mood changes" (p. 16). In other instances the physical problems that an elderly tenant has experienced may be a motivator to seek medical care. When tenants express their concerns or anxieties, professionals should actively listen to identify the nature of these concerns. (Active listening involves receiving information from the elderly tenant in a nonjudgmental manner.)

Housing managers' efforts to get a confused tenant to seek medical attention should recognize the difficulties involved in accurate diagnosis of dementia. General practitioners and internists who have no training in geriatrics are not prepared to diagnose dementia accurately. Housing managers should be knowledgeable concerning either geriatricians or special assessment units in their area that specialize in dementia.

When dementia is suspected, housing managers should also begin to document all tenant behavior that may endanger the safety of the tenant and other tenants (Allen, 1986).

As cognitive decline progresses, housing managers can facilitate the safety of cognitively impaired elderly tenants by increasing the order and predictability of the environment (See Chapter 5). Modifications to make the environment safer include automatic shut-off devices on stoves, handrails, and nonskid bathrooms (Allen, 1986). As deterioration continues, moderately impaired tenants will need supervision and monitoring to ensure that their basic needs are met. During the early stages of the disease, initiation of a telephone "buddy system" can provide a measure of security (Allen, 1986).

According to Allen (1986), the major dangers that may occur for persons suffering from Alzheimer's disease are falls, medication errors, malnutrition, and decreased mobility. As the disease progresses, memory impairment becomes severe. As a result, constant supervision and monitoring are needed.

As housing managers respond to elderly tenants suffering from Alzheimer's disease, their response must take into consideration the special circumstances and resources operating in each situation (Allen, 1986). An elderly tenant with extensive 24-hour support from an elderly spouse may be able to remain in senior housing. In contrast, the tenancy of an individual who has limited assistance or refuses to accept assistance will be jeopardized as mental deterioration declines.Housing managers can perform an important function to educate elderly tenants about normal aging and aging-related changes. For some tenants, fears and stereotypes about dementia may leave tenants who suffer from the disease increasingly isolated and alone. Educational programs can assist tenants in understanding that dementia is not a normal part of aging and can give them strategies for helping persons with dementia (Allen, 1986).

Finally, housing managers and sponsors should develop policies and procedures concerning how to deal with elderly tenants suffering from dementia (Allen, 1986). Policies should provide guidelines for staff concerning their appropriate response, while allowing for consideration of individual factors operating in each situation.

Knowledgeable, patient, and sensitive housing managers and their staff can provide invaluable assistance to tenants and their families as they struggle to deal with the agonizing losses, emotional grief, and physical tasks associated with the progressive loss of cognitive and intellectual abilities.

DEPRESSION AMONG ELDERLY TENANTS

Depression is a common affective or mood disorder among elderly persons. The symptoms of depression, according to Gaylord and Zung (1987), are:

> dysphoric mood, loss of interest, and anxiety. Physical symptoms may include difficulty in falling asleep, loss of appetite and libido, lack of energy, and fatigability. There is often a sense of helplessness and ineffectuality about the present, hopelessness about the future, and a sense of worthlessness and failure about the past (p. 77).

One of the problems in diagnosing depression among the elderly is that its symptoms take on many different forms. According to Cohen (1990), "Depression in particular may wear many different masks in later life: vague physical decline and multiple somatic complaints represent two examples" (p. 361).

Most people associate the symptoms of depression with emotional symptoms such as extreme sadness and crying. For many depressed older persons, however, symptoms are "masked" by other symptoms or complaints. Unless housing managers and social service providers aware of the different manifestations of depression across older persons, depression will not be diagnosed and treated. For some older persons symptoms are expressed primarily as physical, not emotional, complaints. Expressed complaints about physical symptoms that can signal the presence of depression include:

- loss of appetite
- compulsive eating
- inability to sleep
- impairments of digestion or elimination (nausea, heartburn, constipation)
- fatigue
- inability to concentrate

When depression is manifested by only physical symptoms, older persons are frequently not properly diagnosed (Cohen, 1990). The physical symptoms of depression are often attributed to "aging" and normal aging-related changes, making diagnosis of depression very difficult. When depressive symptoms are turned inward, the depressed individual may complain about aches and pains.

In other instances depressive symptoms appear as signs of dementia. Some depressed older persons demonstrate confusion, memory loss, and difficulties in thinking and concentrating. These persons may be misdiagnosed as suffering from dementia. Behavioral manifestations of cognitive decline or clouded thinking may signify the presence of depression. Estimates suggest that between 15% to 20% of depressed older persons experience cognitive impairment associated with their depression (Cohen, 1990).

Sometimes depression among the elderly is characterized by thoughts of worthlessness, belief that the world has little to offer, and the idea that the world is empty. Older persons themselves rarely complain about feeling depressed (Diamond, 1987).

Although the causes of depression are unknown, some older persons become depressed in response to aging-related losses. As a result of losses, elderly persons experience feelings of an inability to control one's life. Older persons who suffer major debilitating chronic illnesses are particularly susceptible to depression (Diamond, 1987).

The failure to diagnose depression leads to missed opportunities for treatment. Because depression can be treated effectively once diagnosed, it is important that housing professionals and social service providers be sensitive to the signs of depression and to encourage depressed older persons to seek treatment.

Prevalence of Depression Among the Elderly

While most experts agree that depression is a fairly widespread problem among the elderly, there is disagreement concerning the exact prevalence rates. Most commonly accepted estimates suggest that between 5% to 15% of community-living elderly are affected by depressive symptoms. In part, disagreements concerning the prevalence rates are due to differences in the criteria used to judge the presence of depression.

The prevalence rates of depression among residents in senior housing are unknown; however, many older tenants demonstrate risk factors that are related to the increased likelihood of being depressed. Elderly tenants who have experienced major role losses, such as death of loved ones; loss of home; loss of income; or chronic, debilitating illnesses may be particularly susceptible to depression. While not all persons who suffer role losses will develop depressive symptoms, these losses may make them vulnerable to depression.

If housing managers recognize the link between feelings of powerlessness and loss of control and depression, they should work to achieve environments that promote control and self-determination among elderly tenants.

REFERRAL FOR MENTAL HEALTH PROBLEMS

Housing managers, social service providers, and health care workers should be aware of the steps underlying successful referral for treatment of mental health problems.

Guidelines for making mental health referrals include (Roff & Atherton, 1989):

1. Actively listen to the concerns expressed. Older persons and their families frequently have difficulty acknowledging that a mental health problem exists. Elderly persons and their families are more likely to share their concerns when the listener conveys an accepting and nonjudgmental attitude.

2. Do not give false reassurance by telling people that "things will be all right".

Rather than false reassurances, older persons need encouragement and support for their decision to seek help. Honest encouragement and support for the decision to seek treatment comes from a belief that growth and change are possible even in advanced old age.

3. Provide accurate information about the options available. To accomplish this, professionals need a thorough knowledge of community services and treatment options for treating the problem.

4. Referrals should be based upon specific knowledge about the community program. Failure to secure adequate information about a treatment program or agency will lead to unsuccessful referrals. The consequences of such unsuccessful referrals are to completely block or frustrate the help-seeking process.

5. Provide information about what will happen in a particular program. Information about exactly what will happen will reduce anxiety that may prevent the elderly tenant from following through with the referral.

6. Provide information about costs of the program and entitlement programs to cover costs. For some elderly tenants, inaccurate perceptions about the financial cost of the program will prevent them from seeking treatment.

7. Follow up to offer support. Answer questions that the elderly and her family may have.

8. Listen for the patient's and family's concerns and respond supportively. (pp. 105-106)

OTHER MENTAL HEALTH CONCERNS
FACING HOUSING MANAGERS

As part of their day-to-day activities, housing managers should strive to create an environment that fosters positive mental health among all elderly tenants. Recognizing that as people age they experience multiple changes and losses, managers in senior housing need to be particularly sensitive and creative in finding ways to enhance positive mental health functioning. From the very beginning they can assist elderly tenants in viewing the move to senior housing as offering increased opportunities to exercise control over the environment and self-determination in their lives. Freedom of choice, opportunities for meaningful social involvement, and rewarding and mutually respectful relationships create a fertile environment for promoting and sustaining good mental health.

In their interactions with elderly tenants, housing managers and social service providers should:

- Treat all elderly tenants with respect
- Acknowledge and accept older persons' feelings and concerns
- Provide meaningful opportunities for social involvement
- Protect elderly tenants' right of self-determination
- Provide resources and opportunities that foster personal growth and development

Housing managers and social service providers should be aware of opportunities for elderly tenants to facilitate their own psychosocial adjustment. The American Association of Retired Persons (AARP) publishes a series of mental health brochures addressing some of the major adjustment issues that older persons confront. (AARP provides multiple copies of the mental health brochures free of charge to interested persons.) Titles in the mental health series include: *So Many of My Friends Have Moved Away or Died, I Wonder Who Else Can Help, If Only I Knew What to Say or Do,* and *Now Where Did I Put My Keys.*

Self-help groups, mutual support groups, and reminiscence groups can also help elderly tenants cope with the changes that have occurred in their lives.

Housing managers' actions in senior housing should be guided by the prinicples of positive mental health or "successful aging." According to Ryff (1986), successful aging is characterized by six dimensions or traits. These are:

1. Self-acceptance
2. Positive relations with others

3. Autonomy
4. Environmental mastery
5. Purpose in life
6. Personal growth

Guided by these goals for successful aging, housing managers will create housing environments that foster successful aging and at the same time personally grow and develop in their own aging process. Whether 30, 40, 50, 60, 70, 80 or beyond, we all need environments that foster our continued growth and development.

CONCLUSION

Housing managers, social service providers, and health care professionals are in ideal positions to help elderly tenants who experience mental health problems to get the help they need. While the prevalence rates of alcohol abuse, dementia, and depression among the elderly are generally not great, the benefits derived from a single older person receiving proper treatment clearly override the efforts to identify and refer elderly tenants to treatment. A sincere belief that the later years offer the potential for satisfaction and enjoyment should underlie all efforts to assist elderly tenants in getting the help they need. Even the oldest, most functionally impaired tenant should be provided opportunities for personal growth and change. Negative attitudes about aging and old age can deprive elderly tenants of opportunities for getting the most enjoyment out of their later years.

Recognizing that the later years can be extremely satisfying and productive, professionals need to be prepared to act when older persons experience psychosocial problems.

10

Working With Special Populations in Senior Housing

THE movement to mainstream special populations into senior housing raises special challenges for housing managers. As populations with special needs—mentally and physically impaired adults—move into senior housing, many housing managers are unprepared to deal with the special issues that emerge. Most managers of senior housing have limited knowledge regarding persons with disabilities.

This chapter examines the legal issues surrounding the integration of special populations into senior housing and presents an overview of the characteristics of special populations as well as strategies for working with disabled adults. Specific attention focuses on the special needs of two populations: mentally retarded adults and persons with a history of mental illness.

THE LEGAL RIGHTS OF HANDICAPPED PERSONS AND INTEGRATION INTO SENIOR HOUSING

Civil rights legislation—the Fair Housing Act, the Rehabilitation Act of 1973 as amended (504), and the Americans with Disabilities

Act—advocate for and protect the rights of all disabled adults. An essential right of all disabled persons protected under civil rights legislation is the right of all persons to have a place to live. Under the Fair Housing Amendments Act of 1988, civil rights protection is extended to persons with disabilities, making it illegal to discriminate against disabled adults in the sale, rental, or financing of dwellings. Under this legislation, a disabled adult is defined as having a physical or mental impairment that substantially limits the individual's ability to carry out one or more major life activities (i.e., walking, hearing, seeing, speaking, working, self-care). The 1988 Amendments also establish design criteria to make multi-family housing built for occupancy on or after March 13, 1991, accessible to and usable by handicapped persons.

The Rehabilitation Act, as amended 504 (Nondiscrimination in Federal Programs) prohibits discrimination by any program receiving federal assistance against persons with disabilities. As a result, excluding disabled adults from federally assisted housing is prohibited. The Americans with Disabilities Act (ADA), signed into law on July 26, 1990, prohibits discrimination against disabled persons in the areas of employment, public accommodations, transportation, and telecommunications. As mandated under the ADA, reasonable accommodations must be made to meet the needs of the disabled.

As a result of these acts at the federal level and legislation at the state level, housing managers cannot discriminate against disabled persons who apply to their housing because of their disabilities. Similarly, housing managers cannot evict disabled or handicapped persons from senior housing because of their disability.

Persons with disabilities protected under the antidiscrimination legislation include all persons with either mental or physical impairments. Because legislation does not exclude elderly persons with disabilities, housing managers may not terminate the tenancy or evict elderly tenants who are physically or mentally impaired—because of their disability. As a result, housing managers find themselves integrating both elderly, elderly handicapped, and younger mentally and physically handicapped persons into senior housing. Further, within senior housing, in order to comply with the mandates of nondiscrimination legislation, housing managers must make reasonable accommodations to house handicapped persons (Falk & Philbrick, 1991).

Many housing managers in their efforts to meet the mandated requirements under law, require help or assistance in understanding how civil rights legislation affects their management practices. Specific areas of concern for housing managers include procedures for screening applicants and terminating tenants.

Screening

In screening applicants for senior housing, managers need to treat all applicants equally. Housing managers may not ask handicapped persons specific questions about their disability. As Falk and Philbrick (1991) state, housing managers should be aware that:

> The only questions that an owner or property manager may ordinarily ask relate to the applicant's ability to meet the requirements of the tenancy imposed on all tenants. A frail elderly tenant (and handicapped applicant), therefore may be asked if she has the financial ability to pay the rent or the ability, with or without assistance to keep her apartment in a clean and safe condition.
> A landlord may not ask, however, about the details of an applicant's medical problems. A landlord may not demand copies of the applicant's medical records or otherwise ask the applicant to waive her right to privacy. (p. 4)

Because traditional screening tools that housing managers use (home visits, landlord references, and credit checks) may discriminate against persons with disabilities, special accommodations may need to be made for disabled persons who lack a rental history. This adjustment may be particularly necessary for deinstitutionalized mental patients. If a handicapped applicant cannot provide a rental history to document his or her ability to meet the requirements under the lease, the manager can ask the applicant to provide other sources of information concerning his or her ability to meet lease requirements. Potential sources for this information, states the U.S. Department of Housing and Urban Development Regional Office I (1991), include, "doctors, therapists, and/ or social service agency personnel, as well as neighbors, relatives, friends or other non-medical sources" (p. 2). Under these circumstances, however, the references should be asked *only* regarding the applicant's ability to meet the terms of the lease.

Terms of the Lease

Because admission to senior housing and continued residence are determined only by a tenant's ability to meet the conditions of the lease, the lease is critical for the management of senior housing. All tenants must be issued the same lease. Special provisions cannot be added or amended to the lease of handicapped tenants. As Falk and Philbrick (1991) state, "A landlord may not condition rental of an apartment on the tenant's signing special lease addenda which obligate her, for example, to receive medical treatment or waive her right to privacy" (p. 6). Because leases must comply with both federal and state antidiscrimination statutes, an attorney should determine that the lease complies with all relevant laws.

Housing managers should pay careful attention to the conditions of the lease. Lease conditions should "oblige tenants to refrain from actions which would threaten the health and safety of other tenants" (U.S. Department of Housing and Urban Development Region I Office, 1991). All tenants need to be made aware that behavior that violates conditions of the lease will jeopardize their continued tenancy. Housing managers must be careful to enforce conditions of the lease for all tenants and document all instances when a tenant's actions threaten the health and safety of other tenants. Housing managers must be careful to provide all tenants with specific information that will help them meet the requirements of the lease.

HOUSING MANAGERS' FEAR AND UNCERTAINTY ABOUT FAIR HOUSING

Many housing managers express fear and uncertainty concerning the consequences of the Fair Housing Act and civil rights legislation prohibiting discrimination against persons with disabilities. Among their fears and concerns are increased discrimination law suits, the impact of the integration of special populations on the quality of life for elderly tenants, and the problems of integrating special populations. Undue levels of fear and anxiety create serious problems that interfere with the capacity of housing managers to do their job.

Under the Fair Housing Act, landlords or property managers must not treat a person differently because he or she has a disability and must make reasonable accommodations to meet the needs of a disabled tenant. More specifically, according to Falk and Philbrick (1991):

> An owner or property manager may not treat an applicant or tenant any differently because that person has a handicap. For example, a landlord may not refuse to rent to an elderly tenant simply because he or she is senile or uses a wheelchair or needs a health care attendant.
>
> In addition, the Fair Housing Act defines discrimination as the failure to make reasonable accommodations for persons with disabilities. For example an elderly tenant with a demonstrated medical need for companionship of a pet may not be denied an apartment even though the management usually has a "no pets" policy. Similarly, the management must assign a parking space near the building to an elderly tenant who has difficulty walking, even though other tenants without disabilities would ordinarily be next in line to get a convenient space (pp. 2-3).

Fear and uncertainty among housing managers about complying with Fair Housing legislation are fueled by several factors. Commonly shared anecdotes concerning the problems that arise when persons with disabilities reside in senior housing describe "horror stories" about housing managers' experiences. Some anecdotes describe the interpersonal conflicts that occur between elderly tenants and younger disabled tenants. It is important to point out, however, that there are no systematic data that support the anecdotes describing problems when special populations are integrated into senior housing. When problems emerge, the reasons for the problems are more likely due to individual or personality factors, not the disability (Karasik, 1989).

For developmentally disabled persons who suffer significant problems associated with their mobility or self-care, certain modifications of the physical environment may be necessary. (Changes or modifications that facilitate disabled persons' ability to function independently are discussed at length in Chapter 5.) Finally, housing managers' fear and uncertainty are due to their negative attitudes about disabled persons and mainstreaming. These negative attitudes are based upon lack of knowledge, suspicion, fear of the unknown, and stereotypes concerning handicapped persons.

Accurate knowledge and understanding concerning persons with disabilities and strategies for integrating disabled persons into the community can significantly reduce fear and uncertainty among housing managers. Housing managers, social service and health care providers must actively seek to rid themselves of stereotypes and misperceptions. Only after professionals honestly address their personal fears and stereotypes can the rights of all persons to live with dignity and independence be advanced.

Successful integration of all groups into senior housing requires basic knowledge about groups of disabled persons, understanding concerning the tremendous diversity within groups of disabled persons, strategies for building a positive social environment for all tenants, and strategies for dealing with tenants who pose a serious threat to the safety of other tenants or cause severe damage to the property.

PERSONS WITH DEVELOPMENTAL DISABILITIES

According to federal statute, the definition of developmental disabilities reflects severe chronic mental or physical impairments that affect the individual's capacity to function in major areas of life activity. By definition, the developmentally disabled adult has three or more substantial limitations in the following areas: self-care, learning, mobility, self-direction, capacity for independent living, and economic self-sufficiency. Under the federal definition, the developmentally disabled adult experienced his or her disability prior to age 22 and will live with the disability throughout his or her adult life. The four most common conditions included under developmental disabilities include: mental retardation, epilepsy, cerebral palsy, and autism. In addition, a variety of other neurological disorders account for approximately 12% of the developmentally disabled population (Kultgen, Guidry, Cohen, Sanddal, & Bourne, 1989).

In the past many persons with developmental disabilities were cared for in institutions. During the 1960s efforts were directed to deinstitutionalize persons with mental retardation and other developmental disabilities. The shift from institutional care to maintaining developmentally disabled adults in the community reflected a major underlying change in treatment philosophy from custodial care to habilitation (Cotten & Spirrison, 1986). The goals of these efforts were to integrate developmentally disabled adults into the community, assist them in obtaining necessary skills for independent living, and enable them to live in the least restrictive environment. As a result, a number of residential alternatives have been developed to serve developmentally disabled adults—skilled nursing facilities (SNFs), intermediate-care facilities (ICFs), intermediate-care facility for the mentally retarded (ICF/MR), personal care homes, group homes, supervised apartment complexes, and shadow supervision (Cotten & Spirrison, 1986). These residential alternatives reflect a continuum of housing alternatives to meet the diverse needs of developmentally disabled adults.

Shadow supervision describes the situation of developmentally disabled adults who are capable of living alone with only minimal supervision (Cotten & Spirrison, 1986). For developmentally disabled adults living in independent housing, the services of a case manager are available to help the person receive needed services. Within this residential category, senior housing provides a possible residential setting for developmentally disabled adults who can live independently in the community. The extent to which senior housing functions as part of the residential continuum serving developmentally disabled adults, however, is unknown.

The tremendous diversity that characterizes the population of the developmentally disabled necessitates a wide range of residential alternatives. While some developmentally disabled adults are severely incapacitated by their disability, the majority do not experience such extreme functional limitations. In fact, the overwhelming majority of these persons do not require extensive help or assistance with personal care and supportive services (Kultgen et al., 1989). Among developmentally disabled persons, more than 90% are either only mildly or moderately limited in some aspects of development (Kultgen et al., 1989). Accurate functional assessment is, therefore, a critical factor in determining appropriate residential placement.

Mental Retardation

By far the largest group of developmentally disabled adults is the mentally retarded. Among mentally retarded adults, great variation exists in their ability to carry out major self-care activities. Persons diagnosed as mentally retarded have lower than average intellectual abilities and capacities. In addition, due to the onset of disability during the period of development, mentally retarded persons experience related deficits in their adaptive functioning. Because of the tremendous variation that exists among persons who are mentally retarded, four categories of impairment are used to describe different ability levels: mild retardation, moderately retarded, severely retarded, and profoundly retarded. Persons who are mildly retarded are capable of performing most adult roles with minimal supervision. As older adults, mildly retarded persons may require support services to help them deal with aging-related changes. According to Kultgen et al. (1989), moderately retarded adults "are able to take care of most of their affairs with support provided by other family members or human service agencies" (p. 6). With aging, moderately retarded adults' reliance on specialized services increases. For severely and profoundly retarded adults, their ability to function is far more seriously impaired. Persons who are severely or profoundly retarded experience major deficits in communication, personal care, and movement. Their needs for long-term care services—supervision, medical attention, and specialized therapies—continue into old age. Many higher functioning mentally retarded adults are capable of independent functioning and self-care and can live in senior housing with either little or no supervision.

Needs of Mentally Retarded Adults

Only limited information exists that describes the needs of mentally retarded adults. The lack of information is due to an inherent bias in research on mental retardation that has focused primarily on mentally retarded children, adolescents, and young adults. Only recently have researchers turned attention to studying elderly mentally retarded adults. Of all age groups, mentally retarded persons between 30 and 50 years of age have received the least amount of attention. As a result, housing, social service, and health professionals have only limited information upon which to base their responses to the needs of middle-aged and elderly mentally retarded persons living in senior housing. The discussion that follows is based primarily on recent work concerning elderly mentally retarded persons.

Mentally retarded adults share the same basic needs and concerns as all adults. In addition, their expectations about what their housing should provide are similar to most persons.

Persons with developmental disabilities expect their home to fulfill the same needs as does anyone else's home. All persons look to the place they call home to meet their needs for physical shelter, meaningful relationships with others, restful and enjoyable leisure time, an opportunity for personal growth and learning, and a respectful attitude from others that assures their dignity and worth as human beings (Summers & Reese, 1986).

Beyond these basic needs, mentally retarded adults evidence tremendous variability in their need for supportive services depending upon their degree of impairment. Supportive services may be provided by family, friends, neighbors, and the formal service system. These services may include emotional support, housing, medical services, supervision, activity programs, and social services. A significant number of mentally retarded adults do not receive services from the formal service system; rather, they rely exclusively on assistance from family, friends, and other sources of informal support to enable them to live independently in the community. Krause (1986) estimated that approximately 40% of mentally retarded adults are not involved at all with the formal support system.

Among those receiving formal services, many receive supportive services from the mental retardation/developmental disabilities (MR/DD) service network. As these mentally retarded adults reach old age, needed formal services may be provided by either the MR/DD network or aging network. Because there is little communication or coordination between the MR/DD and aging network, service delivery and coordination may be a problem for some elderly mentally retarded persons. Further, there is disagreement among experts concerning the best approach to provide formal services to mentally retarded older adults.

Service-Delivery Models and Mentally Retarded Adults

Three service-delivery models have been proposed, each reflecting different assumptions about the best ways to serve mentally retarded older persons. Seltzer and Krause (1987) call these models or approaches:

1. Age integration
2. Generic services integration
3. Specialized service option

The age integration approach provides services to mentally retarded adults of all ages. The generic services integration option integrates elderly mentally retarded adults into existing aging services programs. Included under this approach are both community-based and residential initiatives. Community-based programs for integrating elderly mentally retarded adults include mainstreaming into community programs such as senior citizen centers. Residential programs under this approach include community-living situations mixing mentally retarded older adults with nonretarded older persons.

The generic approach of integrating elderly mentally retarded persons into existing aging services or programs has not been employed frequently. Those programs that have attempted to do so have produced positive results (Seltzer & Krause, 1987). The limited number of such programs, however, limits the generalizability of this conclusion. According to Seltzer and Krause (1987):

> The feasibility and appropriateness of integrating elderly mentally retarded persons into generic senior citizen programs is largely a function of the extent to which the elderly mentally retarded and the elderly nonretarded participants share common characteristics and needs. High functioning elderly mentally retarded persons may be excellent candidates for mainstreaming into generic senior citizen programs. (p. 5)

Overall, information on the integration of either younger mentally impaired and elderly mentally persons into senior housing is extremely limited. The National Survey of Programs Serving Mentally Retarded Persons (Seltzer & Krause, 1987) provides a very brief description of "mixed residential programs" serving elderly mentally retarded with others, such as nonretarded elderly persons with physical handicaps, and persons with emotional problems or history of psychiatric problems. These mixed residential programs serve mentally retarded residents who are either mildly or moderately retarded. Of all types of residential programs surveyed (foster homes, group homes, group homes with nurses, intermediate care facilities for the mentally retarded, apartment programs), integrated or mixed residential programs were least likely to see elderly mentally retarded adults as having special needs. In addition, elderly mentally retarded adults in these settings were most likely to remain in their apartments during the day. This survey, however, provided no information concerning the extent of social integration among elderly nonretarded and mentally retarded adults and elderly.

Research examining the level of social integration of younger disabled in senior housing has noted that most elderly nonhandicapped tenants and younger disabled tenants get along well (Karasik, 1989). When problems occur, the problems were attributed to idiosyncratic or personality conflicts between the younger disabled and elderly tenants—not the disability of the person (Karasik, 1989).

The third approach to service delivery is the specialized service option. This involves special service programs exclusively for elderly mentally retarded adults. Programs and activities are designed for the special abilities of mentally retarded older adults. In contrast to other approaches, this approach segregates elderly mentally retarded adults from all other groups.

The second approach—generic services integration approach—underlies efforts to integrate mentally retarded persons with other elderly nonhandicapped persons.

PERSPECTIVES ON ELDERLY AND DEVELOPMENTALLY DISABLED PERSONS

Recent work addressing approaches to working with both the elderly and persons with developmental disabilities provides insight into the common issues involved in serving both populations.

According to Ansello and Zink (1990), these common issues include: marginality of clientele, issues of family caregiving, contributions by clientele, and heterogeneity. Both elderly and developmentally disabled adults, to varying degrees, are viewed as outside
the mainstream of society. Opportunities to integrate both groups
into society must overcome the prejudices and stereotypes applied to both groups. Second, for many in both groups, the care
received from family caregivers is critical to their overall well-
being. With the aging of both the care recipient and the care
provider, issues facing family caregivers take on renewed importance. Within both groups, increased needs for supportive services place increased stress and strain on the family caregiver
system. Third, within both groups many persons make significant
contributions to the well-being of others. Identifying ways of
optimizing these contributions not only increases their sense of
accomplishment and satisfaction, but also decreases their marginality within the system. Finally, heterogeneity is a critical charac-
teristic of both populations. Increasing heterogeneity is the rule
rather than the exception. Social service providers and housing
managers need to guard against attitudes or interventions that
assume that members of either group become more and more
similar with aging. The "costs" of such assumptions will be missed
opportunities for continued growth and development. For both
groups the philosophy underlying all professional interactions
and programming should be to maximize the individual's growth
and capacity to function.

Opportunities for satisfying use of leisure time are also important
concerns for both groups. As part of the housing manager's role,
efforts should be made to offer a variety of activities that promote a
sense of accomplishment, enjoyment, and pleasure. For some older
mentally retarded tenants who have worked their entire lives in
sheltered workshops and various day programs, adjustment to retirement may pose a special challenge. For others the opportunity to
just take it easy may be particularly appealing. Successful work with
both groups requires an appreciation of these shared issues.

Deinstitutionalized Mental Patients
Integrated Into Senior Housing

Working with tenants who have a history of psychiatric illness presents one of the greatest, most difficult challenges to the management and staff of senior housing. While some chronically mentally ill persons, with proper treatment and medication, adjust satisfactorily to the demands of group living in senior housing, others have tremendous difficulty in adjusting to these demands.

Chronic Mental Health Problems

For many persons suffering from chronic mental illness, access to medical and therapeutic services enables them to live independently in the community. Others who experience difficulty in adjusting to the demands of living in the community have been poorly treated by the mental health treatment system in the past. Factors that complicate the integration of persons suffering chronic mental illness into senior housing include: inadequate treatment systems, their disadvantaged social status (poor, limited education, limited resources), lack of personal and social skills, nonexistent or disrupted social support systems, and negative societal attitudes and stereotypes. These are major barriers that prevent or limit their successful integration into the community (Rathbone-McCuan & Hashimi, 1982).

Community-Based Programs and Resources

A number of community-based programs and resources have been developed to support integration efforts. Efforts to rehabilitate persons with psychiatric disabilities into the community begin with the recognition that many persons with psychiatric disabilities should be integrated into community-living situations (Randolph,

Laux, & Carling, 1987). For those who are capable of living in the community, successful rehabilitation involves providing opportunities to establish meaningful social relationships, the ability to access community services, and involvement in social and leisure activities. To accomplish the goals of rehabilitation for persons with psychiatric disabilities, programs must be individualized to each client's needs. With flexible, individualized programming, many persons with psychiatric disabilities can acquire the necessary skills and support to live successfully in community housing (Randolph et al., 1987).

In the past many persons with chronic mental disabilities have been poorly served by the treatment system. Concepts underlying rehabilitation offer new hope for helping many mentally impaired persons live in the community with dignity and independence. The principles of the rehabilitation approach include: client involvement; personalized living situation and supports; flexible services; commitment to optimal functioning and opportunities for growth and development; access to long-term safe, decent, affordable housing; integration into community life; comprehensive and coordinated services; access to long-term, stable supportive services; development of support systems that include both formal and informal supports; access to a responsive services system; advocacy by the mental health system to overcome problems; and the right to dignity and respect (Randolph et al., 1987).

In communities with mental health programs committed to the principles of rehabilitation, the success of efforts to integrate persons with mental disabilities into senior housing is optimized. For housing managers a collaborative relationship between community mental health programs and housing professionals can be mutually beneficial. In Connecticut a nationally recognized demonstration program involving mental health and housing professionals provides a model for efforts to integrate persons with mental disabilities into subsidized housing. The model program involves a collaborative relationship between a local mental health center and housing authority. The mental health center provides necessary supportive services to disabled persons living in the housing authority's housing complexes. The partnership assures that tenants' needs will be met and that emergency services will be available (Doyle, personal communication, 1991).

Other approaches to meeting the needs of tenants with chronic mental health problems involve the provision of specialized mental health outreach workers in senior housing complexes. In addition, several large housing authorities in Connecticut have secured funding from either their local Area Agency on Aging or community social service agency to hire highly trained mental health outreach workers to provide specialized services to older persons suffering from mental disability.

PSYCHIATRIC DISORDERS

A critical component for housing managers and social service providers to work effectively with persons with mental disabilities is a basic understanding of mental health and psychiatric problems that they encounter. Only a limited effort has been made to assist housing managers in better understanding the various types of mental health problems, related symptoms, and community resources available to serve this population.

The following discussion presents a brief summary of some of the major functional mental health problems. Functional disorders refer to mental health problems that do not have an underlying organic cause and are, therefore, attributable to the person's psychosocial situation. For some persons functional disorders appear early in life, while for others, functional disorders emerge during middle age and old age.

Mental health problems classified as functional disorders include affective disorders (depression, dysphoria, and mania), anxiety disorders, schizophrenia, and paranoid disorders.

Affective Disorders

Depression is characterized by overwhelming feelings of sadness, loss of interest in things, insomnia, lack of energy, inability to concentrate, difficulty in making decisions, irritability, fatigability, and loss of appetite. Coexisting with depression are often feelings of helplessness and inability to do anything about the future, hopelessness, and a sense of worthlessness. Many depressed persons have reoccurring thoughts of death or suicide.

According to the National Mental Health Association (1988), "Depression comes in various forms. Some people experience a single episode of depressive symptoms, and others experience recurrent episodes." For some persons suffering from manic-depression, their moods alternate depressive lows and "manic" highs.

Depression is one of the most prevalent types of mental illness. Once diagnosed, the overwhelming majority of persons suffering from depression can be helped. Treatment for depression involves drug therapy, psychotherapy, and, in some cases, electroconvulsive therapy. The support of caring family and friends who understand the depression makes it much easier for the person to assume his or her normal activities (National Mental Health Association, 1988).

Anxiety Disorders

Anxiety disorders refer to a group of functional disorders characterized by feelings of fear or uneasiness that interfere with the individual's ability to carry out normal activities. Types of anxiety disorders include: anxiety states, phobias, panic disorders, posttraumatic stress disorder, and obsessive-compulsive disorders. People suffering from anxiety disorders experience a wide range of symptoms associated with their condition. These include dizziness, tension, fatigue, sweating, muscle aches, racing heart, numbness or tingling of extremities, upset stomach, cold/clammy hands, jitteriness, and high pulse and/or breathing rate (American Psychiatric Association, 1988a). Overall, persons suffering from anxiety disorders experience recurrent worry and fears concerning their own welfare or that of their loved ones.

Phobic disorders are characterized by irrational fears associated with objects or situations. Persons suffering phobic disorders may progressively curtail their daily activities to avoid the feared or dreaded object or situation. Fear of flying, fear of closed spaces, and fear of public places are examples of common phobias. For many, the desire to avoid the feared object or situation results in progressive isolation.

Panic disorders, according to the American Psychiatric Association (1988a), are characterized by:

intense, overwhelming terror for no apparent reason. The fear is accompanied by at least four of the following symptoms: sweating, heart palpitations, hot or cold flashes, trembling, feelings of unreality, choking or smothering sensations, shortness of breath, chest discomfort, faintness, unsteadiness, tingling, fear of losing control, of dying, or going crazy. (p. 3).

If untreated, persons suffering from panic disorders can become suicidal.

Obsessive-compulsive disorders involve repetitive thoughts or actions with no apparent reasons. In some people obsessions—repeated, unwanted thoughts—are accompanied by ritualistic behaviors (compulsive rituals to deal with obsessive thoughts). In others the disorder is characterized only by the presence of obsessive thoughts. Frequently noted compulsive rituals include cleaning rituals, checking, hoarding, repeating, avoiding, being meticulous, slowness (American Psychiatric Association, 1988b).

Posttraumatic stress disorder (PTSD) is suffered by persons who have experienced severe physical or mental trauma. Most frequently associated with the aftereffects of combat for soldiers, a violent, unexpected event can produce PTSD. Symptoms include nightmares, night terrors, and flashbacks, emotional anesthesia, general anxiety, depression, difficulty concentrating, and survivor's guilt (American Psychiatric Association, 1988a).

Treatment of anxiety disorders involves both drug therapy and psychotherapy. Behavioral therapy is frequently used with persons suffering from phobias and obsessive-compulsive disorders. Medication helps to relieve the symptoms and enables the person to benefit from other types of therapeutic interventions.

Schizophrenic Disorders

Schizophrenic and paranoid disorders are categorized as psychoses. The overall nature of these illnesses involves a loss of touch with reality and disintegration of personality. Persons suffering from schizophrenia experience impairment in thought processes, distorted perceptions, and a distorted sense of self. Symptoms associated with schizophrenia include hallucinations, delusions, and disordered thinking. Hallucinations refer to seeing things, hearing voices, or feeling things that are not present. Delusions refer to recurrent beliefs that are not based upon reality associated with feelings of anxiety or grandeur. Disordered thinking is characterized by disorganized or fragmented thought processes that disrupt logical thinking (National Mental Health Association, 1986). Schizophrenics may display either very little emotionality or inappropriate emotional responses to situations. Communication deficits associated with this disorder include hardly speaking at all or incoherent speech. Treatment involves a variety of different approaches. Some schizophrenics require long-term hospitalization. Others may be treated through short-term or partial hospitalization. A variety of medications are available that lessen some of the symptoms. Medications are most effective in reducing hallucinations, delusions, and disordered thinking (National Mental Health Association, 1986).

Paranoid Disorders

Paranoid disorders are characterized by a delusional state that is frequently accompanied by feelings of being persecuted. As a result, persons suffering from paranoid disorders are convinced that "others" (e.g., the FBI, the other tenants, etc.) are out to get them. While the basis of the delusional system is irrational, the person's delusional system is well developed and follows logically from the initial, irrational premise.

Over time the effects of untreated chronic mental disorders disrupt and erode the social support system of afflicted persons. As a result, many persons who have had a long history of psychiatric problems have fractured or nonexistent social support systems.

COMMUNITY MENTAL HEALTH CENTERS

Community mental health centers provide a resource to assist professionals working with tenants with a history of psychiatric problems (Rathbone-McCuan & Hashimi, 1982). Community mental health centers provide individual and group counseling, case management, day treatment, and emergency services. In some communities mental health centers provide a 24-hour crisis line to deal with suicide threats and serious mental health crises. In addition to providing counseling services, many centers sponsor preventive programs. Outreach to lonely, isolated tenants in senior housing may forestall or prevent the development of serious mental health problems.

The type of service needed—individual or group counseling, day treatment programs, or case management—to maintain persons suffering from a psychiatric illness will vary depending on the nature of the illness. Psychiatric assessment is a critical factor in determining what type of service is most needed to strengthen and support the capacity of the individual to live in independent housing.

Housing sponsors and management should develop a positive working relationship with local mental health centers. Through networking, current information about programs and resources can be exchanged. Further networking provides opportunities for joint planning for program development to address the essential support issues for maintaining chronically impaired adults in independent living situations.

In Connecticut a number of innovative outreach programs have been developed based upon joint planning between community mental health centers and housing sponsors. The Danbury Housing Authority in cooperation with Options, a community mental health center, has developed an agreement to serve chronically impaired persons with services provided by Options. Both individualized case management services and emergency services provide assuredness to the housing authority that the needs of younger mentally disabled persons will be met. The City of New Haven Housing Authority, with funding from the South Central Area Agency on Aging, has a specially designated mental health outreach worker to address the problems of tenants suffering mental health problems. In both instances a local mental health agency provides the housing sponsor with services that support the efforts of mentally impaired persons to live in senior housing. These outreach programs target tenants in senior housing who are experiencing adjustment problems. Typical problems that are addressed through these programs include: isolation, unsafe or unhealthy living conditions, and depression. Tenants have the right to refuse the services offered.

Numerous positive benefits accrue from relationships with community mental health centers. They provide a source of training and information about mental health problems, counseling services to tenants, case management for clients, and, in some communities, emergency services.

A word of caution, however, should be noted about community mental health centers. In many communities these centers are underfunded and understaffed to meet all the needs of the chronically mentally impaired (Rathbone-McCuan & Hashimi, 1982).

ISSUES FOR HOUSING MANAGERS DEALING WITH PERSONS WITH CHRONIC MENTAL HEALTH DISORDERS

Housing managers should be knowledgeable about signs and symptoms of mental health problems and aware of any significant changes that occur in a tenant's behavior that may signal problems requiring intervention. Housing managers and their staff should be particularly aware when problems such as combativeness, inability to care for self, or suicidal talk occur.

Housing managers may not evict a mentally impaired tenant because of his or her bizarre behavior. While this behavior may be troubling to other tenants, if this behavior is not threatening to the health or safety of other residents, it is not sufficient grounds to evict the tenant. In dealing with other tenants, housing managers should provide assurance that the environment is safe, while protecting the confidentiality of the disabled tenant. When housing managers have legitimate concerns about changes in a tenant's behavior, they should express these concerns to the tenant in a nonthreatening manner.

Housing, social service, and health care professionals should get to know the mental health center in their communities. They should take advantage of opportunities to interact with mental health professionals through education, training, and networking and explore options of shared programming addressing mental health needs that are mutually beneficial.

Work with family and friends is also important for helping persons suffering from chronic mental health problems. Families' fears, frustrations, and feelings of loss should be addressed to help the family respond in a caring and effective way to meeting the needs of their troubled relative.

Maintaining open channels of communication between the management and tenants is a particularly important tool for anticipating or avoiding future problems. In the event of a crisis situation, housing managers should be ready to act immediately. For tenants who are experiencing an acute episode of their illness, an immediate referral to an appropriate community mental health resource or program is essential. Access to a 24-hour emergency crisis line through a local mental health center is an invaluable resource to responding to emergency or crisis situations.

MISCONCEPTIONS ABOUT MENTAL ILLNESS

Misconceptions and stereotypes about mental illness create barriers to integrating persons who have mental illnesses into senior housing. The most common misconceptions about mental illness, according to the National Mental Health Association (1987), include:

"People with mental illness will never recover."
"All people with mental illnesses are violent and dangerous to society."
"People who have been treated for a mental illness are unstable and could go 'wild' at any moment."

People with mental illnesses will never recover. Mental illnesses are treatable. With proper treatment, some people with mental illness can and do recover. With proper diagnosis of the cause of the mental illness, a treatment plan can bring improvement and/or recovery. Consequently, persons who have suffered mental illness and have received proper treatment can return to lead normal lives. Prejudice and discrimination against persons with mental illness, however, frequently create obstacles that prevent their integration into the mainstream of society.

All people with mental illnesses are violent and dangerous to society. According to the Mental Health Association (1987), "People with mental illnesses pose no more of a crime threat than do members of the general population." Many persons who are recovering from a mental health problem are likely to be anxious and timid. In fact, persons recovering from mental illness are more likely to be the victims of violent crime. *People who have been treated for a mental illness are unstable and could go "wild" at any moment.* In reality, persons with mental illnesses are not likely to confront others aggressively. More typically, they are likely to withdraw from contact with others. If relapses occur, the symptoms are more likely to develop gradually. Prompt attention to early warning signs can deal with the problem before it becomes serious.

Facts about the reality of mental illness can reduce the fear and uncertainty associated with integrating persons with a history of mental illness into senior housing. It is incumbent upon housing managers to know the facts and to increase elderly tenants' understanding and awareness of mental health problems and issues.

SENIOR HOUSING TENANTS' ATTITUDES

Overall, housing managers should be aware of elderly tenants' attitudes toward persons with disabilities. Because many elderly persons, like people of any age, hold negative stereotypes and prejudices against persons with disabilities, as part of their role, housing managers should educate tenants about disabilities and offer sensitivity training to increase elderly tenants' acceptance of disabled persons.

With the encouragement and support of the housing manager and staff, handicapped or disabled persons can be assured their right to live in the community with dignity and independence. For disabled persons and nondisabled elderly tenants, housing managers should ensure that tenants' needs for physical shelter, meaningful relationships, enjoyable leisure time, personal growth and learning, and respectful attitudes from others are met (Summers & Reese, 1986).

Research examining tenants' attitudes has noted that attitudes toward disabilities vary with respect to the type of disability and across individuals (Karasik, 1989). Some tenants have no problem in accepting others with disabilities, while others hold negative attitudes toward all disabled persons. A study of elderly tenants' attitudes toward living with neighbors with disabilities found that elderly tenants appear most accepting of physically disabled persons (Karasik, 1989). In fact, 78% of elderly tenants reported that "it would be okay" to have a physically disabled person as a neighbor in their housing complex. This figure increased to 98% saying it would be acceptable "as long as the disabled tenant was independent and capable of self care" (Karasik, 1989, p. 31) In contrast, elderly tenants' attitudes were much less accepting of persons with mental impairments. Only 27% of elderly tenants reported that it would be acceptable to have a mentally impaired person move in as their neighbor, while an additional 13% indicated it would be acceptable if the tenant was capable of self care. Among the reasons expressed for not accepting the mentally impaired as neighbors in senior housing were safety fears and disruption of peaceful life-style. As Karasik (1989) reported: one elderly woman said she would not like to have a mentally confused neighbor because, "I'd be afraid they might leave the stove on . . . and start a fire." Another elderly tenant reported an experience that affected her attitude: "I'd had one neighbor . . . always screaming and fighting . . . it was upsetting and frightening. No . . . I wouldn't like that again" (p. 33).

Somewhat similar attitudes were expressed by tenants concerning having a mentally retarded person as a neighbor. Close to 40% reported that having a mentally retarded person live next door would be "okay," while 27% reported that it would be acceptable if the mentally retarded person was completely independent. Several tenants expressed worry and concern about having to take care of a mentally retarded neighbor. As Karasik (1989) relates in the words of a 78-year-old woman, "It's such a worry . . . you wonder how they will manage and worry if you don't drop in enough . . . I feel sorry for someone like that" (p. 34). Twenty-seven percent of tenants, however, reported that it would not be acceptable to have a mentally retarded person living as a neighbor. Their sentiments are expressed by an elderly man's comment, "I wouldn't like it . . . there are other places for them besides here."

Looking specifically at tenants' attitudes toward the integration of younger persons with disabilities into senior housing, whether tenants accepted younger people with disabilities as their neighbors was directly related to their acceptance of a particular disability. Several elderly tenants expressed concerns about whether younger persons with disabilities would be happy "with us old folks." Males, elderly tenants with greater functional limitations, and older tenants were more negative toward the presence of disabled or frail tenants.

Interpersonal conflicts between younger disabled and elderly tenants can arise over issues of territoriality. Particularly as the percentage of younger disabled persons increases, elderly tenants may feel that they are being robbed of their home that was intended for seniors. At a recent meeting, a housing manager of an elderly building with approximately 20% of tenants who are younger disabled reported that elderly tenants are increasingly "bothered" about living with younger disabled tenants. These tenants feel that younger persons do not belong in senior housing. The integration of younger and older handicapped persons into senior housing is facilitated when housing managers have created a warm, socially supportive environment. Sensitivity programs to assist elderly tenants in dealing with their negative attitudes and stereotypes can reduce fear, lack of acceptance, and prejudice against persons with disabilities.

CONCLUSION

Legal, demographic, public policy, and social imperatives demand that housing managers, social service providers, and health care professionals be prepared to work with special populations in senior housing. Adequate preparation should entail knowledge about the needs of persons with disabilities, sensitivity to the individual and shared needs of all persons, effective linkages between housing and social service professionals providing essential services to disabled persons, and the capacity to develop innovative social programs that integrate disabled persons into the life of the complex.

Many housing managers fail to realize that persons with disabilities have needs similar to those of all persons. Housing managers' efforts in managing housing, state Summers and Reese (1986), should address all persons' needs for "physical shelter, meaningful relationships, enjoyable leisure time, personal growth and learning, and respectful attitudes from others" (p. 121). Managers who have fostered a positive social climate in their housing will be better able to integrate persons with special needs into senior housing. The challenge to achieve the successful integration of persons with disabilities is great for housing managers. Many have responded to the challenge by creating innovative social service programs that provide essential services to ensure the success of disabled persons' efforts to be integrated into the community.

In the future more and more innovative solutions will emerge as partnerships are formed with professionals from the DD/MR and mental health fields that seek successful programs to support disabled persons in the community. Housing managers can serve as pioneers in forwarding the success of the movement to integrate special populations into senior housing.

11

Housing Managers, Social Service
Providers, and Health Care
Professionals Working Together

Due to the dramatic changes that have impacted on the senior
housing industry—increased numbers of vulnerable elders, greater
unmet needs, increased extensiveness of support needs, and greater
difficulty in mobilizing support services—there is a growing need
for housing managers, social service providers, and health care
professionals to work together to meet the needs of vulnerable or
at risk elderly tenants. This chapter explores (a) the underlying
reasons why alliances are becoming increasingly important, (b)
the barriers that inhibit collaboration and cooperation, and (c) the
basic elements for successful collaboration.

THE IMPORTANCE OF ALLIANCES AMONG
HOUSING, SOCIAL SERVICE, AND
HEALTH CARE PROFESSIONALS

The increased importance of alliances among housing, social
service, and health care professionals is based upon several sig-

nificant trends that affect elderly tenants' need for and ability to access essential community-based support services. These trends include the unprecedented numbers of vulnerable elderly tenants who need community-based services to remain living independently in the community; the fragmentation and lack of coordination of existing programs and services at the federal, state, and local levels; a shift in the locus of the long-term care delivery system to serve impaired elderly in the least restrictive environment (Chellis, Seagle, & Seagle, 1982; Lawton, 1980; Newman, 1985; U.S. Senate Special Committee on Aging, 1990); a schism between long-term care and housing and social service policies (Newman, 1990; Tilson & Fahey, 1990); cutbacks in appropriations for housing and supportive services (U.S. Senate Special Committee on Aging, 1990); and changes in Fair Housing policies enabling increasingly impaired or functionally dependent tenants to remain in senior housing.

As a result of these trends, more and more moderately to severely impaired elderly tenants requiring community-based long-term care services are living in senior housing. Despite their increased need for supportive services, however, public policies have yet to address how the needs of this vulnerable or at risk group can be met. Currently the lack of comprehensive public policies integrating housing, social services, and health care, growing fiscal restraints, and lack of a system for delivering community-based long-term care leave many elderly tenants without essential services and place them at increased risk of premature institutionalization (Tilson & Fahey, 1990). The present situation has created tremendous pressures on housing managers, social service providers, health care professionals, frail elderly tenants and their families because mechanisms for responding to the ever increasing needs do not exist.

Given the lack of institutional support for the delivery of services to functionally impaired elderly tenants, as the numbers of functionally impaired tenants increase, housing professionals alone are unable to respond to these emerging support needs.

Efforts to assist elderly tenants can succeed only if housing, social service, and health care professionals work together to improve elders' ability to access essential community services. The purpose of alliances involving housing, social service, and health care professionals is to develop innovative approaches to meeting the support needs of vulnerable or at risk elderly tenants. Through the formation of partnerships, limited resources can be utilized in the most efficient and effective ways to meet older persons' shelter/service needs (Tiven & Ryther, 1986). Creation of these partnerships must transcend traditional professional boundaries and barriers that have prevented housing, social service, and health care professionals from working together by defining a common goal to address the support needs of elderly tenants. The call for partnerships recognizes that many problems have prevented cooperation and collaboration among these groups. As elderly tenants' needs for support increase, however, there is an urgent need to develop resourceful solutions to meet these growing needs. In addition, as the numbers of elderly tenants who are unable to carry out essential activities of daily living continue to grow, the importance of partnerships will increase over the next decades (Biegel, Shore, & Gordon, 1984; Sheehan, 1988a, 1989).

SOCIAL SUPPORT AND SOCIAL NETWORK THEORY: A THEORETICAL PERSPECTIVE ON PARTNERSHIPS

A growing body of literature describes the importance of social support in the lives of individuals. Social support is linked positively to physical and psychological health. Social support or assistance helps the individual either directly or indirectly to cope more effectively with life stresses.

Due to the positive effects of social support in individuals' lives, a variety of interventions to strengthen social support in the lives of vulnerable populations have been proposed (Biegel et al., 1984; Froland, 1982; Hooyman, 1983). These interventions are aimed at mobilizing and strengthening support through the activation of the helping network—the informal, formal, and quasi-formal systems. While ideally all components of the social support system work together to maximize the assistance that vulnerable older persons receive, in most cases, support is received from only the informal support system. If the informal support system is limited or nonexistent, many vulnerable individuals do not receive the support they need.

Both institutional and personal barriers operate to prevent the mobilization of support networks for vulnerable elders. Institutional factors that prevent older persons from receiving essential support services include restrictive eligibility requirements, costly services, bureaucratic red tape, impersonal services, fragmentation of services, or lack of services in a geographic location (Hooyman, 1983). Personal factors can also prevent tenants from being able or willing to access available services. These factors include: lack of knowledge about services, personal and familial values that stress independence and self-reliance, and fear of seeking help outside the family (Springer & Brubaker, 1984).

As a result, either personal or institutional factors have a direct impact on whether or not an elderly tenant receives the support or assistance that he or she needs. As more and more elderly tenants become increasingly vulnerable and experience the risk of nursing home placement, the need for partnerships or alliances has become increasingly clear (Biegel et al., 1984; Cantor & Little, 1986; Clayton, Schmall, & Pratt, 1985; Froland, 1982).

Partnerships may be designed to include a wide variety of persons and groups. In response to identified needs among elderly tenants, alliances may take a number of different forms or shapes. Membership in these partnerships may include both professionals and nonprofessionals, professionals and family members, elderly tenants and professionals, and so on. Regardless of the form that these partnerships take, alliances will only be successful if they are based upon: (a) a thorough knowledge and understanding of the strengths, weaknesses, and interactions that characterize all components of the support system; (b) a sensitive understanding of how members in support networks view their role; and (c) recognition of the barriers that inhibit cooperation and collaboration among the different support group members (Froland, 1982; Hooyman, 1983; Sheehan, 1987).

The overall goals of such partnerships are to enhance the delivery of care to vulnerable or at risk older persons and to mobilize the helping network on their behalf. Because these partnerships involve new roles for professionals —advocate, consultant, coordinator organizer, and facilitator (Biegel et al., 1984)—housing managers, social service providers, and health care professionals must be prepared to define their roles in much less traditional ways. Rather than developing all interventions focused directly on elderly tenants, alliances may seek to provide support to family members to assist their efforts in helping elderly tenants or increase coordination among community-based agencies to increase the flow of information to tenants. Other examples of creative partnerships include building a volunteer network within religious institutions to respond to elderly tenants' needs or convening informational programs about services designed to breakdown barriers that prevent older persons from utilizing formal services.

BARRIERS TO ALLIANCES OR PARTNERSHIPS

The formation of alliances or partnerships involving housing, social service, and health care professionals is particularly challenging because it must overcome numerous barriers that prevent these groups from working together. The major reasons why building partnerships may be particularly challenging include lack of understanding and awareness of the other professional groups involved; previous negative experiences involving either housing, social service or health care professionals that have produced distrust or misperceptions; lack of clarity regarding role expectations and role boundaries of housing managers, social service providers, and health care professionals; lack of a common forum for addressing critical issues; lack of shared channels of communication; lack of shared training around issues of elderly tenants and support services; and noninterfacing networks of professional groups.

First and foremost, housing managers, social service providers, and health care professionals frequently do not understand the unique challenges and problems that the other professional groups face. For effective partnerships professionals must be sensitized to understanding the unique situation that each group faces in dealing with the problems of vulnerable elderly tenants. Social service and health care professionals must understand the responsibility of the housing manager for assuring the safety and well-being of all elderly tenants. Housing managers must understand that social service and health professionals strive to assure their elderly clients with the best quality care.

Lack of understanding among housing managers, social service providers, and health care professionals occurs frequently when a housing manager decides that it is necessary to relocate an impaired tenant to a more supportive residential environment. Problems, in part, arise around relocation decisions if housing, social service, and health care professionals do not accurately understand the role and responsibilities of the other professionals involved. Anecdotes from both housing managers and social service and health care professionals about relocation frequently describe intense conflicts. Housing managers will often complain about an "overzealous" social service or health care professional who attempted to thwart their efforts to relocate a tenant who was a threat to the safety of other residents. Similarly, social service or health professionals complain when a housing manager "arbitrarily" decides to "evict" one of their clients. In part, potential conflicts around issues of termination or relocation can be reduced if housing managers, social service, and health care professionals work together.

Working together, housing, social service, and health care professionals can achieve increased understanding and appreciation of the roles that the other plays. As a result, previous negative experiences may be replaced by positive experiences when housing managers, social service, and health professionals work together cooperatively. Through dialogue and joint planning, professionals serving functionally impaired elderly tenants can also increase their capacity to more effectively serve impaired older persons.

TYPES OF PARTNERSHIPS SERVING VULNERABLE ELDERLY TENANTS

Successful alliances or partnerships can take many forms and approaches. According to Froland (1982), these range from "establishing communication linkages, carrying out systematic planning processes, and providing forums for community involvement, to a more ambitious structuring of community-wide networks" (p. 252).

Among some of the most promising activities around which alliances can be built are joint community planning, shared training, forums for community involvement, and personal networking. Positive shared experiences bringing together housing, social service, and health care professionals can forge a common bond in efforts to meet vulnerable elders' needs for supportive services. Opportunities to express common concerns, frustrations, and satisfactions provide occasions to understand the demands involved in their respective roles. Joint forums for addressing the policy and service-delivery issues that confront these professionals provide opportunities for identifying unmet needs.

Bringing housing professionals together with social service and health care professionals is a relatively new idea. Our own experiences bringing together housing managers and social service and health professionals in a federally funded model continuing education training program, the Elderly Renters Project, helped sensitize us to both the barriers that operate against such initiatives and the benefits derived from successful linkages (Sheehan, 1991). As implementation of the training program progressed, we listened to initial resistance expressed by some housing specialists about the idea of joint training sessions. Concerns expressed, in part, reflected perceptions of the difficulties involved in bringing together these different groups. Because most continuing education programs train housing managers with housing managers, social service professionals with other social service professionals, and so on, the idea of bringing together both groups was seen by some as either "risky" or "foolish." The problem, however, in separate training for housing, social service, and health care professionals is that it does nothing to increase mutual understanding among these critical professional groups who must interact frequently concerning the problems of at risk elderly tenants.

Despite some initial skepticism, our experiences conducting the Elderly Renters Project training program, Managing for Success: Problem Solving Strategies for Working with Frail Elderly Renters, provided convincing support for the benefits of this approach. Through the training, participants identified common problems that they encounter, shared their unique perspectives when problems associated with aging in place emerge, and enjoyed opportunities for dialogue and networking with others. Shared educational experiences are a positive first step in moving toward more comprehensive, systematic attempts to build alliances involving housing, social service, and health care professionals.

BASIC ELEMENTS FOR SUCCESSFUL
ALLIANCES COLLABORATION

As previously discussed, alliances or partnerships can take many different forms and target different components of vulnerable elders' social support networks. The basic elements necessary for successful collaboration include:

- A thorough knowledge and understanding of how social networks operate
- Respect for the roles that the members in the partnership play
- Open channels of information exchange and communication

Without these basic elements, any attempt to form alliances or partnerships will be unsuccessful.

Lack of knowledge about the complex, dynamic interactions that characterize social networks leaves professionals with misconceptions concerning how their actions, the actions of other professionals, family members, and others influence the quality of support or assistance available to vulnerable elders. Housing managers and social service and health care professionals need to understand how change in one component of the support system reverberates throughout the entire support system.

The interdependence among the informal, formal, and quasi-formal support systems is frequently ignored or overlooked. Examples of this interdependence include changes in policies to retain more vulnerable elderly in senior housing increase tenants' needs for support services; termination of homemaker services to a functionally impaired elderly tenant creates a tenuous situation regarding his or her ability to continue living in senior housing; social service professionals' belief that tenants in senior housing are better off than other elderly living in the community will limit community-based services available to them; housing managers' negative attitudes toward families will reduce the amount of support that family members provide; or social service providers' assumption that all tenants who need services will avail themselves of needed services will limit outreach to isolated elderly tenants.

Through training and education, housing, social service, and health care professionals can increase their understanding of social support in the lives of elderly tenants. Increased understanding will provide professionals with insights into the most effective ways for assisting elderly tenants.

Second, successful partnerships or alliances require knowledge and understanding concerning the roles that housing managers, social service providers, and health care professionals play in the lives of elderly tenants. Confusion regarding professional roles and boundaries can lead to conflicts. Clear descriptions concerning the roles and responsibilities of professionals help to:

- Identify the unique contributions that each partner can make in the alliance
- Delineate overlapping areas of responsibilities
- Identify the limitations of responsibility

The task of defining the role of housing managing is particularly challenging because the role is undergoing a transition. Mechanisms for achieving understanding of roles include joint training, dialogue, and networking. Opportunities to interact with professionals serving elderly tenants include participation in professional networks that cross professional disciplines. Housing managers should participate actively in local aging organizations, such as Councils on Aging, home care advisory groups, and the like, while social service and health care professionals should serve on advisory boards and planning committees for senior housing complexes.

Despite differences among roles, all members of the partnership must maintain the same professional standards and ethical principles in their work.

Finally, other efforts should be directed at improving the exchange of information through joint newsletters, community forums, and conferences dealing with housing and supportive services.

The impetus for developing alliances may come from professionals in the housing, social service, or health care fields. Our own observations have documented a variety of partnerships that have emerged as a result of actions from each of the three sectors. A few examples will illustrate some of the successful partnerships that link together housing and supportive services to meet vulnerable elderly tenants' needs.

A housing manager of a large urban senior housing complex approached a local home care agency with concerns about the growing numbers of functionally impaired tenants living in her complex. After much discussion, the decision was made to locate a case manager from the home care agency in the complex for 3 days each week.

Because more than half of the elderly tenants in the complex were clients of the home care agency, the arrangement to provide case management services on-site was beneficial to both the elderly tenants living in the complex and the home care agency.

A second example of a partnership to meet vulnerable elders' needs came about through concerns of a town's elderly outreach worker. The outreach worker noted that increased numbers of isolated elders resided in the town's senior housing complexes. The outreach worker, together with the Executive Director of the local housing authority, developed a proposal to fund a part-time outreach worker to serve elderly tenants in senior housing complexes. The proposal was funded with municipal funds. The presence of the outreach worker has reduced the problem of isolation among many elderly tenants.

A Volunteer Tutor Program was initiated through joint planning by a housing manager and local school board. The program recruits volunteers from the senior housing complex and provides volunteers to several local schools.

Local home health care aides have been recruited from a local senior housing complex. A local home care agency provides the training. The home health aide program provides a source of reliable, dependable home health aides, while at the same time providing a source of income to low-income elderly tenants. Frequently trained home health care aides provide services to tenants who live in their senior housing complex.

These are only a few examples of how innovative programs or partnerships can be established when housing, social service, and health care professionals come together to more effectively serve the needs of elderly tenants.

CONCLUSION

Reflecting about the developments that have occurred in senior housing during the past 20 years, I have found it increasingly clear that there have been marked changes in what we know as senior housing. Increased acceptance of the view that senior housing should be more than shelter alone has altered significantly the role of housing managers. As a result of the changing view of senior housing, housing managers, social service providers, and health care professionals have become pioneers in charting new directions for senior housing.

During the 1990s the challenges for professionals serving elderly tenants in senior housing will be increasingly addressed. Through increased education, training, and sensitivity to the needs of elderly tenants, issues concerning the quality of life of elderly tenants will continue to be addressed.

Appendix A

Assessment of Independent Living Skills

Assessment of Independent Living Skills

Instructions

The Assessment* includes 20 routine living skills or conditions. The 20 skills or conditions are further delineated as being Critical or Contributory factors in determining the status of a person's ability to live independently. Critical factors relate directly to lease requirements and immediate health and safety conditions. If a resident's skill level in any of these critical factors is inadequate, serious consideration should be given to a supervised service-intensive living arrangement. If a person's skill level is inadequate in more than one or two contributory factors, an independent living situation may not be advisable. The availability and appropriateness of supportive services and a willingness on the part of the individual to accept services are factors that must be considered.

The Assessment should not be treated or used as an inflexible absolute from which there is no appeal. All factors and extenuating circumstances must be discussed and weighed in order to afford the fairest assessment. Participation of the resident in the decision-making process should be routinely encouraged and supported whenever possible.

The assessment is a tool intended to be used as an outline for evaluation and recertification of elderly and handicapped housing applicants and tenants. Often these evaluations are conducted by one person and, as a consequence, are somewhat subjective. Nevertheless, if the Assessment is used, the evaluator will have covered all important aspects of independent living skills with the applicant or tenant thereby providing a more comprehensive appraisal of abilities and needs.

*The Assessment is adapted from guidelines developed by the Human Services Department of the Public Housing Agency of the City of Saint Paul (PHA), partially based on materials presented in: *A Social Work Guide for Long-Term Care Facilities.* (DHEW Publication No. (ADM) 75-177, Printed 1975), developed by the National Institute of Mental Health. Reprinted with permission from the Human Services Department of the Public Housing Agency of the City of Saint Paul.

Assessment of Independent Living Skills

CRITICAL AND CONTRIBUTORY	ADEQUATE PERFORMANCE	INADEQUATE PERFORMANCE	UNABLE TO JUDGE
1. MEAL PREPARATION DIET	☐	☐	☐
2. HOUSEKEEPING	☐	☐	☐
3. MOBILITY	☐	☐	☐
4. PERSONAL CARE: TOILET	☐	☐	☐
5. PERSONAL CARE: MEDICATIONS	☐	☐	☐
6. TIME, PLACE, PERSON ORIENTATION	☐	☐	☐
7. PERSONAL HEALTH & WELFARE PLANNING & DECISION MAKING	☐	☐	☐
8. PRESENCE & EFFECT OF ANXIETY, DEPRESSION, PHOBIAS, PARANOIA	☐	☐	☐
9. ALCOHOL/DRUG ABUSE	☐	☐	☐
10. ROUTINE SAFETY AWARENESS	☐	☐	☐
11. SHOPPING CAPABILITIES	☐	☐	☐
12. FINANCIAL	☐	☐	☐
13. TRANSPORTATION	☐	☐	☐
14. PERSONAL CARE: BATHING	☐	☐	☐
15. PERSONAL CARE: DRESSING	☐	☐	☐
16. PERSONAL CARE: GROOMING	☐	☐	☐
17. PERSONAL HABITS AND CHARACTER TRAITS RELATING TO GROUP LIVING CAPABILITIES	☐	☐	☐
18. CAPABILITY TO MAINTAIN INTERPERSONAL RELATIONSHIPS	☐	☐	☐
19. COMMUNICATION CAPABILITIES HEARING, SIGHT, SPEECH, WRITING	☐	☐	☐
20. TELEPHONE COMMUN- ICATION CAPABILITY	☐	☐	☐

Items 1–10: CRITICAL SKILLS

Items 11–20: CONTRIBUTORY SKILLS

CRITICAL AND CONTRIBUTORY SKILLS

ADEQUATE	INADEQUATE	BASIS OF JUDGMENT EVIDENCE
1) Able to prepare adequate meals independently. Eats without assistance.	Requires extensive regular assistance with meals or refuses to prepare or eat adequate meals.	
2) Does housekeeping alone or with occasional help.	Cannot maintain acceptable level of cleanliness and refuses assistance or assistance is not available.	
3) Is mobile without any aids or with mechanical aids (wheelchair, cane, walker).	Requires extensive regular assistance to carry out routine living functions such as in and out of wheelchair, dressing, or toilet.	
4) Toilet-Cares for self at toilet completely. No incontinence.	Has no control over bladder or bowels.	
5) Medications - Is responsible for taking medications in correct dosages at correct times without assistance.	Requires daily or excessive supervision of medications for more than short periods of time.	
6) Has little or no difficulty with time, place, person orientation.	Severely disoriented in regard to time, place, and person.	
7) Able to fully participate in planning and exercises good judgment in decision making in matters relating to personal health and welfare.	Capacity for planning and decision-making requires considerable help from others or memory disorientation is sufficient to warrant daily or around the clock nursing supervision.	
8) Free of symptoms such as anxiety, depression, phobias, or paranoia, or these symptoms may be present in a mild form but do not significantly hinder daily functioning.	May have moderate or severe symptoms pointing to a danger to self or others.	

CRITICAL AND CONTRIBUTORY SKILLS

ADEQUATE	INADEQUATE	BASIS OF JUDGMENT EVIDENCE
9) Use of drugs or alcohol is not abusive and has not caused disturbances.	Frequently under the influence of alcohol and/ or drugs. Is displaying disruptive behavior. Is not maintaining own health and apartment.	
10) Is aware of and practices routine safety measures.	Refuses to practice or is frequently unaware of normal safety precautions.	
11) Obtains groceries and other items needed for daily living.	Cannot or will not obtain food and other necessary items.	
12) Manages financial matters independently. Writes and cashes checks, pays rent and bills, collects and keeps track of income.	Incapable of handling financial matters. Has or needs guardian. Refuses assistance or assistance is not available.	
13) Travels independently on public transportation or drives own car or arranges own travel.	Requires extensive assistance with transportation or help in obtaining transportation for medical appointments or adequate transportation is not available.	
14) Bathing: Bathes self (tub, shower, or sponge bath) without help.	Cannot or will not wash self. Refuses assistance or assistance is not available.	
15) Dressing: Dresses, undresses, and selects clothes from own wardrobe with no or very minor assistance.	Needs major assistance with dressing and assistance is not available.	
16) Grooming: (Neatness, hair, nails, hands, face, clothing). Adequately dressed and groomed.	Needs regular assistance or supervision in grooming.	

CRITICAL AND CONTRIBUTORY SKILLS

ADEQUATE	INADEQUATE	BASIS OF JUDGMENT EVIDENCE
17) Is free of disturbing or disabling behavior patterns, character traits, and personal habits that affect capacity for group living. Or has mildly disturbing traits and habits that do not significantly impair capacity for group living.	Exhibits severely disturbing behavior, traits, or habits requiring considerable supervision or counseling. May be incapable of conforming to socially acceptable standards of group conduct. Behavior traits or habits create severe problems in group living.	
18) Maintains satisfactory interpersonal relationships with family, friends, and other residents. Or, may be having minor problems or may be becoming less active in sustaining relationships.	Needs considerable or excessive counseling, encouragement, and stimulation. Less apt than formerly to be interested or concerned about others. Refuses or is unable to maintain interpersonal relationships.	
19) Is able to speak and hear, read, and write with little or no difficulty that may necessitate use of electronic or mechanical aids.	Has severe impairments of communication faculties. has excessive difficulty in understanding and/or being understood.	
20) Is able to dial at least a few well-known phone numbers and is able to converse understandably. May need electronic aid.	Cannot or will not use phone at all, or refuses to have phone even though necessary for health and safety.	

Appendix B

Computerized Case
Management Assessment

EXAMPLE OF COMPUTERIZED WELLNESS PROFILE

FUNCTIONAL ASSESSMENT

Resident Name: Smith, Sally   Resident ID #00000001

Functional Assessment Score: 0 = least independent; 5 = most
  independent

Assessment Dates:	4/25/87	08/26/87	01/11/88	02/09/88
Apartment Maintenance	4	4	4	3
Bathing	4	4	4	4
Expressive Communication	4	4	5	5
Receptive Communication	5	4	4	4
Continence (urinary)	5	4	4	2
Emotional Status	4	4	4	3
Grooming and Dressing	5	4	4	3
Hearing	5	5	5	5
Meal Preparation	5	4	3	2
Medications	5	4	4	3
Mobility	4	4	4	4
Money Management	5	4	3	3
Orientation	5	5	4	4
Physical Health	5	4	4	3
Shopping	5	4	4	3
Social Activities	5	5	3	3
Support Network	4	5	4	4
Toileting	5	5	4	3
Travel	4	4	4	2
Vision	4	4	4	3
ACUITY	4.6	4.25	3.6	3.3

RECOMMENDATIONS

Independent -	4.25	&	4.6	Action Plan:
Assisted Living -	3.6	&	3.3	
Nursing Home -	Not applicable			

References

Adams, R. G. (1985-1986). Emotional closeness and physical distance between friends: Implications for elderly women living in age-segregated and age-integrated settings. *International Journal of Aging and Human Development, 22,* 55-76.

Aging in place: "Indicators" trigger assessment (1989, October). *Housing the Elderly Report, 10,* 1-2.

Alexander, F., & Duff, R. (1988). Social interaction and alcohol use in retirement communities. *The Gerontologist, 28,* 632-636.

Allen, D. G. (1986). *Alzheimer's disease.* Madison: Center for Health Sciences of the University of Wisconsin-Madison.

Ambrogi, D. M. (1990). Nursing home admissions: Problematic process and agreements. *Generations, XIV* (Supplement), 72-74.

American Psychiatric Association. (1988a). *Anxiety disorders.* Washington, DC: Author.

American Psychiatric Association. (1988b). *Obsessive-compulsive disorders.* Washington, DC: Author.

Amis, K. (1987). *The old devils.* New York: Summit Books, Simon and Schuster.

Ansello, E. F., & Zink, M. B. (1990, February). The Partners Project: Targeting community-based research and education on aging developmental disabilities. Paper published in the *Proceedings of the 1990 Lifelong Learning Research Conference,* Arlington, Virginia.

Antonucci, T. C. (1990). Social supports and social relationships. In R. H. Binstock & L. K. George (Eds.), *Handbook of aging and the social sciences* (3rd ed., pp. 205-226). New York: Academic Press.

Atkinson, R. (1984). Substance abuse and abuse in later life. In R. Atkinson (Ed.), *Alcohol and drug abuse in old age* (pp. 2-17). Washington, DC: American Psychiatric Press.

Bauwens, S. (1986). *Drug and alcohol abuse among older people.* Madison: Center for Health Sciences of the University of Wisconsin-Madison.

Beck, A. T., Steer, R. A., & McElroy, M. G. (1982). Relationships of hopelessness, depression and previous suicide attempts to suicidal ideation in alcoholics. *Journal of Studies of Alcoholism, 43,* 1042-1046.

Benedict, R. (1977). Integrating housing and services of older persons. In W. Donahue, M. Thompson, & D. Cumen (Eds.), *Congregate housing for older persons: An urgent need, a growing demand* (pp. 21-26). Washington, DC: Government Printing Office.

Bennett, R. (1973). Living conditions and everyday needs of the aged with specific reference to social isolation. *Journal of Aging and Human Development, 4,* 179-198.

Bevis, L., & Bing, L. (1961). *Senior housing golden age center program.* Washington, DC: Government Printing Office.

Biegel, D. E., Shore, B. K., & Gordon, E. (1984). *Building support networks for the elderly: Theory and application.* Beverly Hills, CA: Sage.

Bienenfeld, D. (1987). Alcoholism in the elderly. *American Family Physician, 36,* 163-169.

Blank, T. O. (1991). *Working with frail elderly renters: The physical environment.* Storrs: University of Connecticut.

Borgatta, E. F., Montgomery, R. J. V. & Borgatta, M. L. (1982). Alcohol use and abuse, life crisis events, and the elderly. *Research on Aging, 4,* 378-408.

Brody, E. M. (1985). Parent care as a normative family stress. *The Gerontologist, 25,* 19-29.

Brody, J. (1982). Aging and alcohol abuse. *Journal of American Geriatric Society, 30,* 123-126.

Brody, J. (1984). Remarks during general discussion panel. In G. Maddox, L. Robins, and N. Rosenberg (Eds.), *Nature and extent of alcohol problems among the elderly* (pp. 319-320). NIAAA Research Monograph No. 14, DHHS Publication No. (ADM) 84-1321. Washington: Government Printing Office.

Butterfield, D., & Weidemann, S. (1987). Housing satisfaction of the elderly. In V. Regnier & J. Pynoos (Eds.), *Housing the aged: Design directives and policy considerations* (pp. 133-152). New York: Elsevier North-Holland.

Cantor, M., & Little, V. (1986). Aging and social care. In R. Binstock & E. Shanas (Eds.), *Handbook of aging and the social science* (pp. 745-781). New York: Van Nostrand Reinhold.

Carp, F. (1987). The impact of planned housing: A longitudinal study. In V. Regnier & J. Pynoos (Eds.), *Housing the aged: Design directives and policy considerations* (pp. 43-79). New York: Elsevier North-Holland.

Carstensen, L. (1987). Age-related changes in social activity. In L. Carstensen, & B. Edelstein (Eds.), *Handbook of clinical gerontology* (pp. 222-237). New York: Pergamon.

Cavanaugh, J. C. (1990). *Adult development and aging.* Belmont, CA: Wadsworth.

Chappell, N. L., & Badger, M. (1990). Social isolation and well-being. *Journal of Gerontology: Social Sciences, 44,* 169-176.

Charatan, F. (1985). Depression and the elderly: Diagnosis and treatment. *Psychiatric Annals, 5,* 313-316.

Chellis, R., Seagle, J., & Seagle, B. (1982). *Congregate housing for older persons: A solution for the 1980s.* Lexington, MA: Lexington Books.

Christensen, D., & Cranz, G. (1987). Examining physical and managerial aspects of urban housing for the elderly. In V. Regnier & J. Pynoos (Eds.), *Housing the aged: Design directives and policy considerations* (pp. 105-132). New York: Elsevier North-Holland.

Christenson, M. A. (1990). *Aging in the designed environment.* New York: Haworth.

Clayton, D., Schmall, V., & Pratt, C. (1985). Enhancing linkages between formal services and the informal support systems of the elderly. *Gerontology and Geriatrics, 5,* 3-11.

Cohen, F., Bearison, D. J., & Muller, C. (1987). Interpersonal understanding in the elderly. *Research on Aging, 9,* 79-100.

Cohen, G. D. (1990). Psychopathology and mental health in the mature and elderly adult. In J. E. Birren, & K. W. Schaie (Eds.), *Handbook of the psychology of aging* (pp. 359-374). New York: Academic Press.

Cotten, P. D., & Spirrison, C. L. (1986). The elderly mentally retarded (developmentally disabled) population: A challenge for the service delivery system. In S. J. Brody, & G. E. Ruff (Eds.), *Aging and rehabilitation: Advances in the state of the art* (pp. 159-187). New York: Springer.

Cranz, G. (1987). Evaluating the physical environment: Conclusions from eight housing projects. In V. Regnier & J. Pynoos (Eds.), *Housing the aged: Design directives and policy considerations* (pp. 81-104). New York: Elsevier North-Holland.

Diamond, R. J. (1987). *Depression among older people.* Madison: Center for Health Sciences of the University of Wisconsin-Madison.

Diehl, P. (1990). *Workbook for developing a Personal Care Sponsor Statement for the residents of Bacon Congregate Housing, Hop River Homes, Welles Country Village, Westerleigh.* Vernon, CT: Elderly Housing Management.

DiStefano, A. F., & Ashton, S. J. (1986). Rehabilitation for the blind and visually impaired. In S. J. Brody & G. E. Ruff (Eds.), *Aging and rehabilitation: Advances in the state of the art* (pp. 203-217). New York: Springer.

Ekerdt, D., DeLabry, L., Glynn, R., & Davis, R. (1989). Change in drinking behaviors with retirement: Findings from the Normative Aging Study. *Journal of Studies on Alcohol, 50,* 347-353.

Evans, D. A., Funkenstein, H. H., Albert, M. S., Scherr, P. A., Cook, N. R., Chown, M. J., Hebert, L. E., Hennekens, C. H., & Taylor, J. O. (1989). Prevalence of Alzheimer's disease in a community population of older persons: Higher than previously reported. *Journal of the American Medical Association, 262,* 2551-2556.

Faletti, M. (1984). Human factors research and functional environments for the aged. In I. Altman, M. P. Lawton, & J. Wohlwill (Eds.), *Elderly people and the environment* (pp. 195-239). New York: Plenum.

Falk, G. W., & Philbrick, J. (1991). *Working with frail elderly renters: Legal issues for housing managers.* Storrs: University of Connecticut.

Feingold, E., & Werby, E. (1990). Supporting the independence of elderly residents through control over their environment. *Journal of Housing for the Elderly, 6,* 25-32.

Finlayson, R. E. (1984). Prescription drug abuse in older persons. In R. M. Atkinson (Ed.), *Alcohol and drug abuse in old age* (pp. 62-70). Washington, DC: American Psychiatric Press.

Fisk, C. F. (1988, March). Address. *Surgeon General's Workshop: Health Promotion and Aging.* Proceedings. Social Security Administration Publication No. 11-11542. Baltimore, MD: Social Security Administration.

Froland, C. (1982). Community support systems: All things to all people. In D. Biegel, & A. Naparstek (Eds.), *Community support systems and mental health* (pp. 253-266). New York: Springer.

Gaitz, C., & Baer, P. (1971). Characteristics of elderly patients with alcoholism. *Archives of General Psychiatry, 24,* 372-378.

Gaylord, S. A., & Zung, W. W. K. (1987). Affective disorders among the elderly. In L. L. Carstensen, & B. A. Edelstein (Eds.), *Handbook of clinical gerontology* (pp. 76-95). New York: Pergamon.

Hamden Housing Authority. (1990). *Personal Care Sponsor Statement.* Hamden, CT: Author.

Harel, Z., & Harel, B. (1978). On-site coordinated services in age-segregated and age-integrated public housing. *The Gerontologist, 18,* 153-158.

Hellman, L. H. (1990). Senior resident vs. senior highrise—Liability for transferring elderly residents. In L. Pastalan (Ed.), *Aging in place: The role of housing and social supports* (pp. 101-105). New York: Haworth.

Hiatt, L. (1987). Designing for the vision and hearing impaired. In V. Regnier, & J. Pynoos (Eds.), *Housing the aged: Design directives and policy considerations* (pp. 341-372). New York: Elsevier North-Holland.

Hofland, B. (1990). Value and ethical issues in residential environments for the elderly. In D. Tilson (Ed.), *Aging in place: Supporting the frail elderly in residential environments* (pp. 241-271). Glenview, IL: Scott, Foresman.

Holshouser, W. L. (1985). Aging in place: The demographic and service needs of elders in urban public housing. Boston, MA: Citizens Housing and Planning Association.

Hooyman, N. (1983). Social support networks in services to the elderly. In J. Whittaker, & J. Garbarino and Associates (Eds.), *Social support networks: Informal helping in the human services* (pp. 133-164). Hawthorne, NY: Aldine.

Hurt, R., Finlayson, R., Morse, R., & Davis, L. (1988). Alcoholism in elderly persons: Medical aspects and prognosis of 216 inpatients. *Mayo Clinic Proceedings, 63,* 753-760.

Kane, R. A., & Kane, R. L. (1981). *Assessing the elderly: A practical guide to measurement.* Lexington, MA: Lexington Books.

Karasik, R. J. (1989). *Social interaction and integration among elderly, frail elderly, and younger handicapped tenants of public senior housing.* Unpublished master's thesis, University of Connecticut, Storrs.

Krause, M. W. (1986). *Long-term care issues in mental retardation.* Paper presented at the National Institute of Child Health and Human Development and the Kennedy Foundation Conference, Mental retardation: Accomplishments and new frontiers, Bethesda, MD.

Kultgen, P., & Guidry, J., Cohen, G. J., Sanddal, N., & Bourne, B. (1989). *Enhancing services for mentally retarded/developmentally disabled residents in nursing homes.* Kansas City, MO: UMKC Institute for Human Development University Program Affiliated Program for Developmental Disabilities and Columbia, MO: Office of Continuing Education and Extension.

Kuypers, J. A., & Bengston, V. L. (1983). Toward competence in the older family. In T. H. Brubaker (Ed.), *Family relationships in later life* (pp. 211-228). Beverly Hills, CA: Sage.

Lawton, M. P. (1975). *Planning and managing housing for the elderly.* Monterey, CA: Brooks-Cole Publishing.

Lawton, M. P. (1980). *Environment and aging.* Monterey, CA: Brooks/Cole.

Lawton, M. P. (1983). Environment and other determinants of well-being in older persons. *The Gerontologist, 23,* 349-357.

Lawton, M. P. (1985). The elderly in context: Perspectives from environmental psychology and gerontology. *Environment and Behavior, 17,* 501-519.

Lawton, M. P., Greenbaum, M., & Liebowitz, B. (1980). The lifespan of housing environments. *The Gerontologist, 20,* 56-64.

Lawton, M. P., Moss, M., & Grimes, M. (1985). The changing service needs of older tenants in planned housing. *The Gerontologist, 25,* 258-264.

Lawton, M. P., & Nahemow, L. (1973). Ecology and the aging process. In C. Eisdorfer, & M. P. Lawton (Eds.), *Psychology of adult development and aging* (pp. 619-674). Washington, DC: American Psychological Association.

Manton, K. G. (1984, March). The future growth of the long-term care population: Projection based on 1977 National Nursing Home Survey and the 1982 Long-Term Care Survey. In U.S. Congress, Senate, Special Committee on Aging, *Development in Aging Report* (Vol. 1.).

Manton, K. G., & Liu, K. (1984). *The future growth of the long-term care population: Projections based on the 1977 national nursing home survey and the 1981 long-term care survey.* Washington, DC: Health Care Financing Administration.

Moore, G. T. (1986, November). *The environment in interactional and transactional theories of environment and aging.* Paper presented at the 39th Annual Meeting of the Gerontological Society of America, Chicago.

Moos, R. H., Lemke, S., & David, T. G. (1987). Priorities for design and management in residential settings for the elderly. In V. Regnier & J. Pynoos (Eds.), *Housing the aged: Designing directives and policy considerations* (pp. 179-206). New York: Elsevier North-Holland.

Morris, J., Gutkin, C., Ruchlin, H., & Sherwood, S. (1990). Aging in place: A longitudinal example. In D. Tilson (Ed.), *Aging in place: Supporting the frail elderly in residential environments* (pp. 25-52). Glenview, IL: Scott, Foresman.

Morse, R. (1988). Substance abuse among the elderly. *Bulletin of the Menniger Clinic, 52,* 259-269.

National Center for Health Statistics. (1986, September). *Current estimates from the National Health Interview Survey.* DHHS Pub No. (PHS) 86-1588, Hyattsville, MD: Author.

National Institute on Aging Eighth Report to Council on Program Fiscal Year 1986. (1986). Washington, DC: U.S. Department of Health and Human Services.

National Mental Health Association. (1986). *Schizophrenia.* Alexandria, VA: Author.

National Mental Health Association. (1987). *Stigma: A lack of awareness and understanding.* Alexandria, VA: Author.

National Mental Health Association. (1988). *Depression.* Alexandria, VA: Author.

Newman, S. (1985). Housing and long term care: The suitability of the elderly's housing to the provision of in-home services. *The Gerontologist, 25,* 35-40.

Newman, S. (1990). The frail elderly in the community: An overview of characteristics. In D. Tilson (Ed.), *Aging in place: Supporting the frail elderly in residential environments* (pp. 3-24). Glenview, IL: Scott, Foresman.

Osgood, N. J. (1987). The alcohol-suicide connection in late life. *Postgraduate Medicine, 81,* 379-384.

Parmelee, P. A., & Lawton, M. P. (1990). The design of special environments for the aged. In J. E. Birren & K. W. Schaie (Eds.), *Handbook of the psychology of aging* (pp. 464-488). San Diego, CA: Academic Press.

Pastalan, L. A. (1990). Designing a humane environment for the frail elderly. In D. Tilson (Ed.), *Aging in place: Supporting frail elderly in residential environments* (pp. 273-286). Glenview, IL: Scott, Foresman.

Patterson, C. (1990). Meeting the demands of a graying America. *Journal of Property Management* (reprint).

Perry, D., Kurland, J., & Citron, H. (1989). *More than a place to live: A training manual for managers of housing and health care facilities for the elderly.* Baltimore, MD: National Health Publishing.

Philbrick, J., Sheehan, N. W., & Blank, T. (1991). *Managing for success: Problem solving strategies in working with frail elderly renters* (90AT0425/01). Washington, DC: Administration on Aging.

Pruzinsky, E. W. (1987). Alcohol and the elderly: An overview of problems in the elderly and implications for social work practice. *Journal of Gerontological Social Work, 11,* 81-93.

Pynoos, J. (1987). Housing the aged. Public policy at the cross-roads. In V. Regnier, & J. Pynoos (Eds.), *Housing the aged: Design directives and policy considerations* (pp. 25-40). New York: Elsevier North-Holland.

Pynoos, J. (1990). Public policy and aging in place: Identifying the problems and solutions. In D. Tilson (Ed.), *Aging in place: Supporting the frail elderly in residential environments* (pp. 167-208). Glenview, IL: Scott, Foresman.

Randolph, F. L., Laux, B., & Carling, P. J. (1987). *In search of housing: Creative approaches to financing integrated housing.* (Monograph Series on Housing and Rehabilitation in Mental Health). Boston, MA: Boston University, Center for Psychiatric Rehabilitation.

Rathbone-McCuan, E., & Hashimi, J. (1982). *Isolated elders.* Rockville, MD: Aspen Systems.

Regnier, V. (1987). Design directives: Current knowledge and future needs. In V. Regnier, & J. Pynoos (Eds.), *Housing the aged: Design directives and policy considerations* (pp. 3-24). New York: Elsevier North-Holland.

Rodin, J., Timko, C., & Harris, S. (1985). The construct of control: Biological and psychosocial correlates. *Annual Review of Gerontology and Geriatrics, 5,* 3-55.

Roff, L. L., & Atherton, C. R. (1989). *Promoting successful aging.* Chicago: Nelson Hall.

Rook, K. (1984). The negative side of social interaction: Impact on psychological well-being. *Journal of Personality and Social Psychology, 46,* 1097-1108.

Ryff, C. (1986, November). *The failure of successful aging research.* Paper presented at the Annual Meeting of the Gerontological Society of America, Chicago.

Ryther, B. (1987). *Aging in place . . . training for managers.* Washington, DC: Council of State Housing Agencies and the National Association of State Units on Aging.

Schlesinger, L., & Morris, J. (1982). Characteristics of public housing clients. In J. Morris, S. Sherwood, & L. Schlesinger (Eds.), *Serving the vulnerable elderly in Massachusetts: The role of the Commonwealth's Home Care Corporations* (pp. 101-108). Report submitted to the Massachusetts Department of Elder Affairs.

Seltzer, M. M., & Krause, M. W. (1987). *Aging and mental retardation: Extending the continuum.* Washington, DC: American Association on Mental Retardation.

Sheehan, N. W. (1986a). Aging of tenants: Termination policy in public senior housing. *The Gerontologist, 26,* 505-509.

Sheehan, N. W. (1986b). Informal support among the elderly in public senior housing. *The Gerontologist, 26,* 171-175.

Sheehan, N. W. (1987). "Aging in place" in public senior housing: Past trends and future needs. *Home Health Care Services Quarterly, 8,* 55-77.

Sheehan, N. W. (1988a). *The Caregiver Information Project: Establishing an information network for family caregivers* (No. 90AT0309/01). Final Report submitted to the Administration on Aging, U. S. Department of Health and Human Services, Washington, DC.

Sheehan, N. W. (1988b). The dynamics of helping behavior in congregate housing. *Activities, Aging and Adaptation, 12,* 13-26.

Sheehan, N. W. (1989). The Caregiver Information Project: A mechanism to assist religious leaders to help family caregivers. *The Gerontologist, 29,* 703-706.

Sheehan, N. W. (1991). *The Elderly Renters Project: A model training program for housing managers and social service providers* (90AT0425/01). Washington, DC: Administration on Aging.

Sheehan, N. W., & Mahoney, K. (1984). *Connecticut's elderly living in public senior housing.* Report submitted to the Gerontological Society of America, Washington, DC.

Spring, J. C., & Kuehn, N. H. (1990). Legal services. In A. Monk (Ed.), *Handbook of gerontological services* (pp. 420-449). New York: Columbia University Press.

Springer, D., & Brubaker, T. (1984). *Family caregivers and impaired elderly: Minimizing stress and maximizing independence.* Beverly Hills, CA: Sage.

Struyk, R. J. (1987). Housing adaptations: Needs and practices. In V. Regnier, & J. Pynoos (Eds.), *Housing the aged: Design directives and policy considerations* (pp. 259-276). New York: Elsevier North-Holland.

Suggs, P. K., Stephens, V., & Kivett, V. R. (1987). Coming, going, remaining in public housing: How do the elderly fare? *Journal of Housing for the Elderly, 4,* 87-104.

Summers, J., & Reese, M. (1986). Residential services. In J. Summers (Ed.), *The right to grow up* (pp. 119-148). Baltimore, MD: Paul H. Brookes.

Sykes, J. T. (1989). *Housing managers care managers.* Madison: Center for Health Sciences of the University of Wisconsin-Madison.

Taylor, S. E., & Brown, J. D. (1988). Illusion and well-being. A social psychological perspective on mental health. *Psychological Bulletin, 103,* 193-210.

Tenant Assistance Program of the Massachusetts Housing Finance Agency (1991). *Alcohol abuse: A guide for managers for the elderly.* Boston: Massachusetts Housing Finance Agency.

Thompson, M. (1982). Enriching environments for older persons. In R. Chellis, J. Seagle, & B. Seagle (Eds.), *Congregate housing for older persons: A solution for the 1980s* (pp. 1-12). Lexington, MA: D. C. Health.

Tilson, D., & Fahey, C. J. (1990). Introduction. In D. Tilson (Ed.), *Aging in place: Supporting the frail elderly in residential environments* (pp. xv-xxxiii). Glenview, IL: Scott, Foresman.

Timko, C., & Moos, R. H. (1990). Determinants of interpersonal support and self-direction in group residential facilities. *Journal of Gerontology: Social Sciences, 45,* S184-192.

Tiven, M., & Ryther, M. (1986). *State initiatives in elderly housing: What's new, what's tried and true.* Washington, DC: Council on State Housing Agencies and National Association of State Units on Aging.

Tobias, C., Lippmann, S., Pary, R., Oropilla, T., & Embry, C. (1989). Alcoholism in the elderly: How to spot and treat a problem the patient want to hide. *Postgraduate Medicine, 86,* 67-79.

Tobin, S. S., & Toseland, R. W. (1990). Models of services for the elderly. In A. Monk (Ed.), *Handbook of gerontological services* (pp. 27-51). New York: Columbia University Press.

U.S. Department of Health and Human Services. (1987, September). Report to Congress by Task Force on Long-Term Care Policies. Washington, DC.

U.S. Department of Housing and Urban Development (1983, August). Memo from the U.S. Department of Urban Development Boston Regional Office, Boston, MA.

U.S. Department of Housing and Urban Development Boston Regional Office, Region 1 (1991, April). Memo concerning screening tenants and complying with civil rights laws. Boston, MA.

United States House of Representatives Select Committee on Aging. (1989). *The 1988 National Survey of Section 202 Housing for the Elderly and Handicapped.* Washington, DC: Government Printing Office.

United States Senate, Special Committee on Aging. (1990). Special Committee on Aging, *Developments in aging: 1989* (Vol.1). Washington, DC: U.S. Government Printing Office.

Wolfsen, C. R., Barker, J. C., & Mitteness, L. S. (1990). Personalization of formal social relationships by the elderly *Research on Aging, 12,* 94-112.

Name Index

215

Subject Index

About the Author

Nancy W. Sheehan, Ph.D., is an Associate Professor in the School of Family Studies, University of Connecticut, Storrs, and a Faculty Associate of the Travelers Center on Aging. Her most recent scholarly activity has examined the role of informal support in the lives of elderly persons. Specific areas of research include: informal support and helping among elderly tenants in senior housing, family caregiving, and the role of the church in providing aging supportive services. Most recently she has been involved in developing a model training program for housing managers and social service providers to assist them in responding to the needs of elderly tenants who have aged in place. In addition, she is investigating the impact of the placement of Resident Services Coordinators in federally assisted senior housing on elderly tenants' well-being. She has coauthored *Managing for Success: Problem Solving Strategies for Working with Frail Elderly Tenants*. Her publications examining elderly housing issues have appeared in *The Gerontologist, Journal of Gerontological Social Work*, and *Home Health Care Services Quarterly*.